OPHTHALMOLOGY COLORING BOOK

Learn and enjoy coloring the components of the Eye.

INTRODUCTION

Ophthalmology is a medical specialty that encompasses the study of the eye's anatomy, physiology, and diseases. It involves the comprehensive diagnosis and treatment of various eye conditions, ranging from minor irritations to severe vision-threatening ailments.

In this field, ophthalmologists are highly trained medical doctors who possess specialized expertise in identifying and managing eye disorders. They employ a diverse array of techniques and tools such as medications, surgical interventions, and corrective lenses to ensure optimal eye health for their patients.

TABLE OF CONTENT

The eye Anatomy …………………………… 5

Eye mouvment ……………….……………… 15

Strabismus ………….…………………… 18

The Human Retina…………………………… 22

Retinopathy ……………………………….. 33

   Macular Degeneration…………………… 35

   Diabetic Retinopathy…………………... 42

   Retinal Detachment …………………… 48

Visual System ….………………………….. 53

Binocular Vision …….…………………… 54

Visual Pathways ……………………… 56

Midbrain ………………………………… 60

Lacrimal Gland ………………………… 62

Cornea ………………………………… 68

Corneal Abrasion …….………………… 71

Ischemic Optic Neuropathy …………… 72

Optic Neuritis………………………….... 76

Glaucoma ……………………………… 82

Cataract ………………………………… 90

Pterygium …………………………… 97

Pinguecula …………………………… 101

Ptosis …………………………………… 105

Myopia ……………………………… 111

Hyperopia ……………………………119

Astigmatism …………………………125

The eye Anatomy:

The eye is an organ of remarkable complexity that enables us to perceive the world around us. It is comprised of various components, each with its own specialized function. For instance, the cornea serves as the transparent outer layer of the eye, responsible for directing incoming light onto the retina. Conversely, the iris plays a role in regulating light intake by adjusting the size of the pupil.

Additionally, other crucial elements include the lens, which aids in focusing light onto the retina, and the optic nerve, responsible for transmitting visual information from the retina to the brain. Familiarizing oneself with ocular anatomy proves indispensable in both diagnosing and managing a wide array of eye ailments.

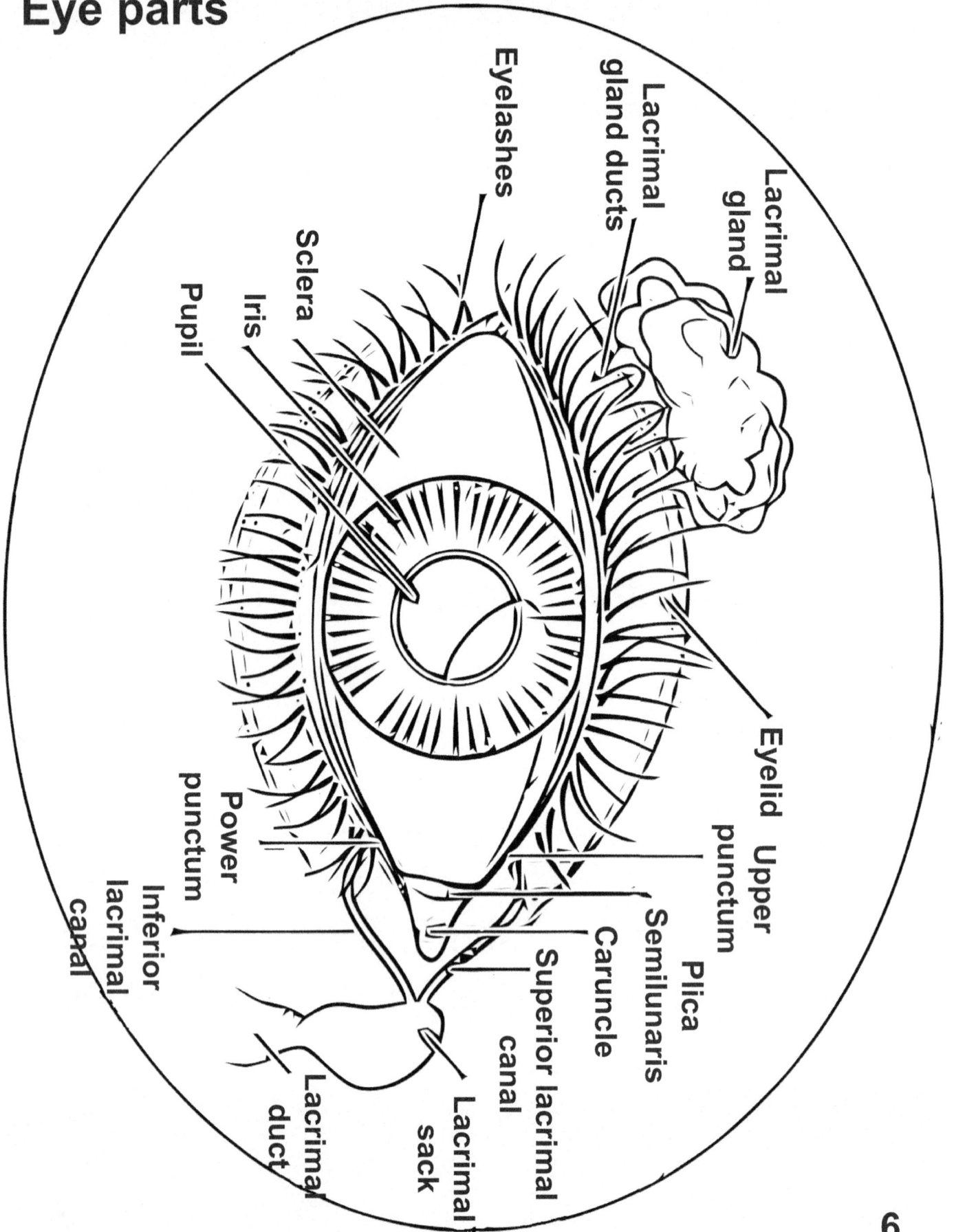

Eye parts

Lacrimal gland ducts

Lacrimal gland

Eyelashes

Sclera

Iris

Pupil

Eyelid Upper punctum

Power punctum

Inferior lacrimal canal

Lacrimal duct

Lacrimal sack

Superior lacrimal canal

Caruncle

Plica Semilunaris

<u>The cornea and sclera</u> are vital components that collaborate to safeguard and sustain the eye's structure.

The cornea acts as a transparent, domed layer that shields the front of the eye. It serves as a barrier against debris, such as dirt and dust, while permitting light to enter the eye. Conversely, the sclera constitutes the outer white layer of the eye. This layer offers support and protection to the fragile internal structures. Additionally, it aids in maintaining the eye's form and contributes to its distinctive aesthetic.

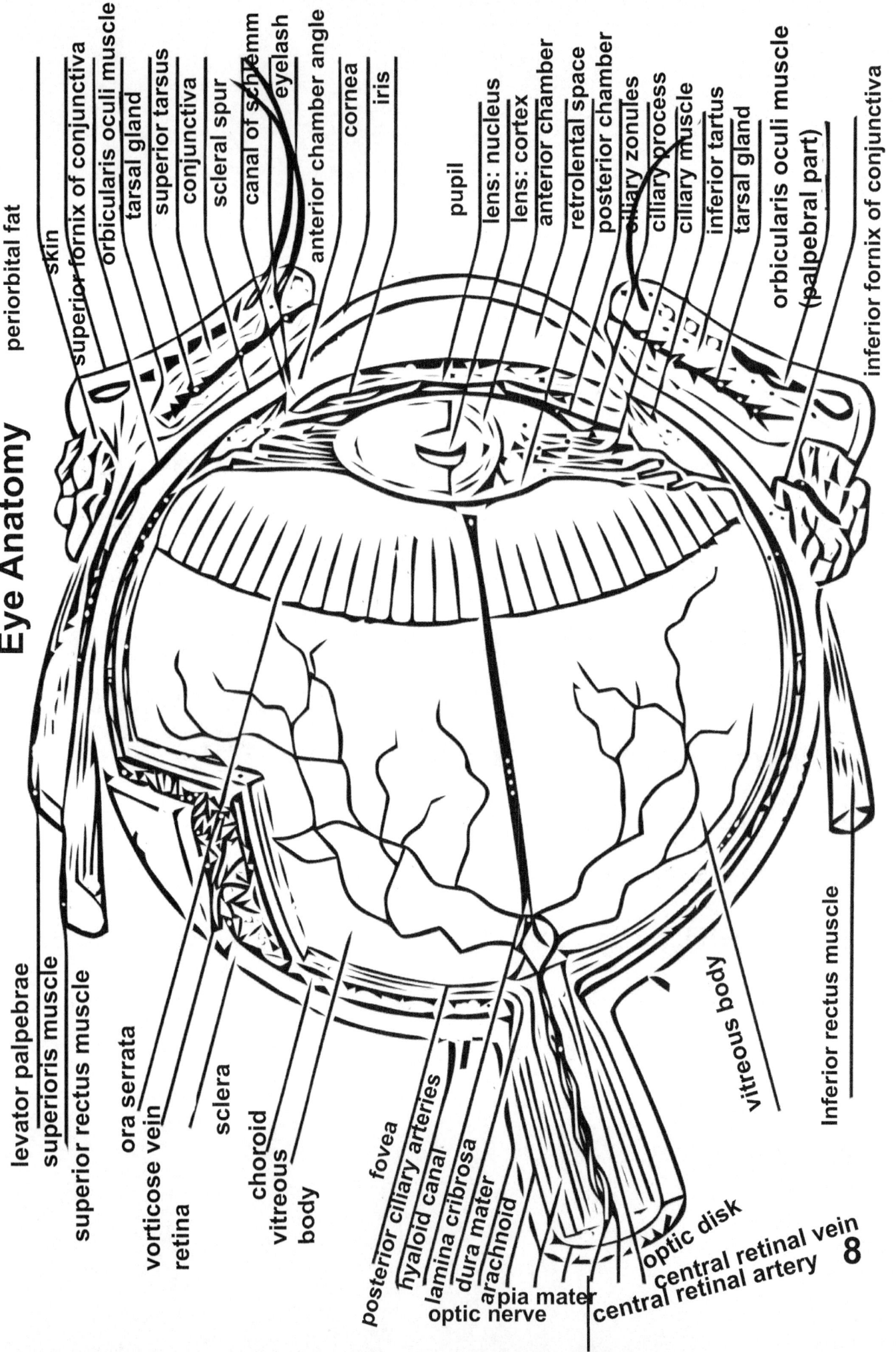

Eye Anatomy

periorbital fat

skin

superior fornix of conjunctiva

orbicularis oculi muscle

tarsal gland

superior tarsus

conjunctiva

scleral spur

canal of Schlemm

eyelash

anterior chamber angle

cornea

iris

pupil

lens: nucleus

lens: cortex

anterior chamber

retrolental space

posterior chamber

ciliary zonules

ciliary process

ciliary muscle

inferior tartus

tarsal gland

orbicularis oculi muscle (palpebral part)

inferior fornix of conjunctiva

levator palpebrae superioris muscle

superior rectus muscle

ora serrata

vorticose vein

retina

sclera

choroid

vitreous body

fovea

posterior ciliary arteries

hyaloid canal

lamina cribrosa

dura mater

arachnoid

pia mater

optic nerve

optic disk

central retinal vein

central retinal artery

vitreous body

Inferior rectus muscle

8

<u>The iris and pupil</u> have a vital role in regulating the amount of light that enters the eye. The iris, which is the part of the eye with color, contains muscles that control the size of the pupil. In bright light, the iris contracts to make the pupil smaller, limiting the amount of light entering the eye. Conversely, in dim light, the iris expands to make the pupil larger, allowing more light to enter.

Moreover, emotional or physiological stimuli can also cause changes in pupil size. When we experience fear or excitement, our pupils can dilate involuntarily. Additionally, certain medications have an impact on pupil constriction or dilation. Understanding how the iris and pupil work together to regulate light is crucial for comprehending the intricacies of our visual system.

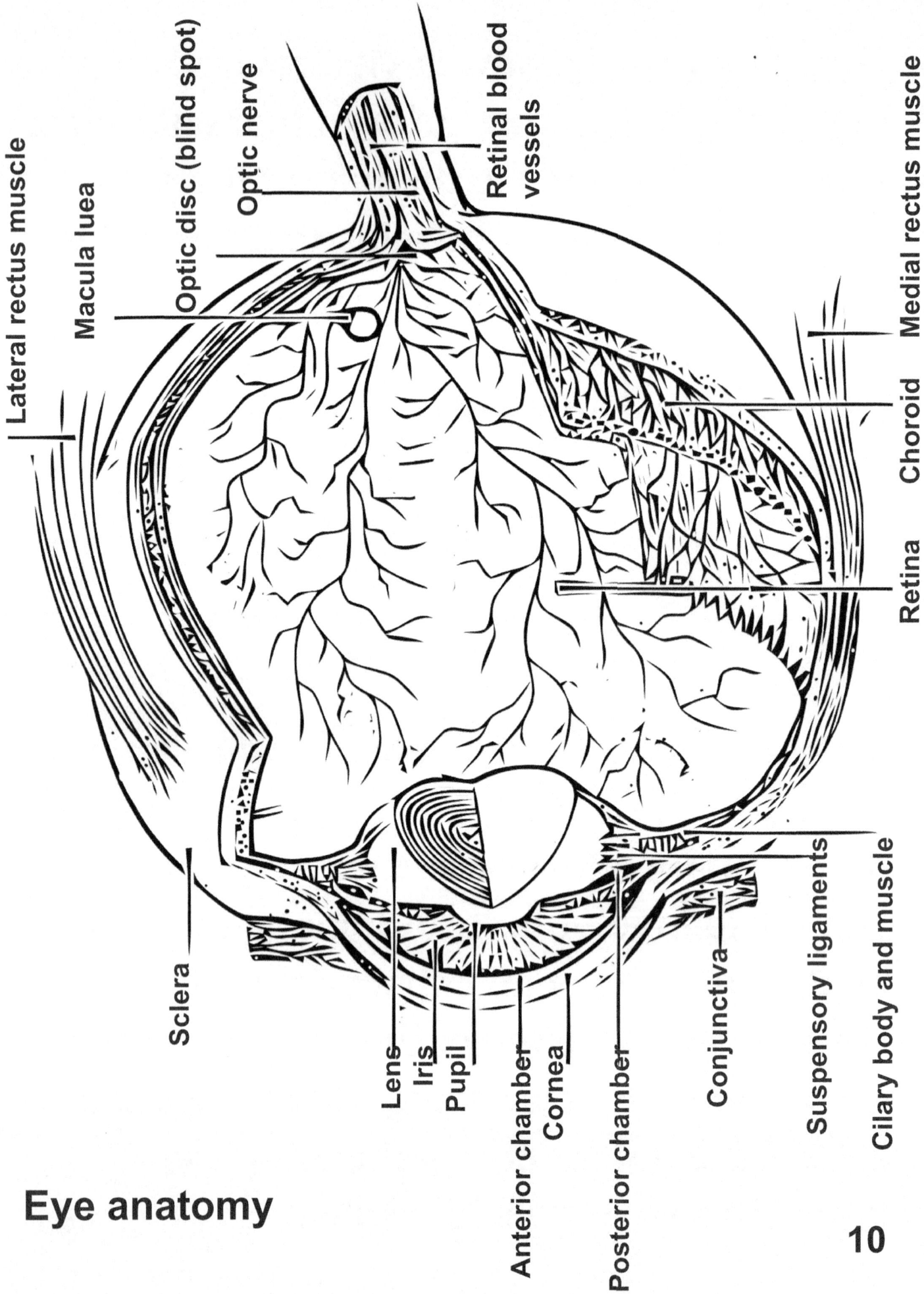

Lateral rectus muscle

Macula luea

Optic disc (blind spot)

Optic nerve

Retinal blood vessels

Medial rectus muscle

Choroid

Retina

Sclera

Lens

Iris

Pupil

Anterior chamber

Cornea

Posterior chamber

Conjunctiva

Suspensory ligaments

Cilary body and muscle

Eye anatomy

10

<u>The lens</u> is an essential component of the eye that works in conjunction with the ciliary muscles to focus incoming light onto the retina. When we shift our focus to near objects, the ciliary muscles contract, causing the lens to thicken and refract light more effectively. Conversely, when we look at distant objects, the ciliary muscles relax, allowing the lens to flatten and decrease its refractive power.

This adjustment of the lens shape based on distance is known as accommodation. Accommodation plays a vital role in our ability to see objects clearly at varying distances without relying on external visual aids like glasses or contact lenses. It is a remarkable function of the eye that ensures our vision remains sharp and adaptable.

Anatomy of the eyeball

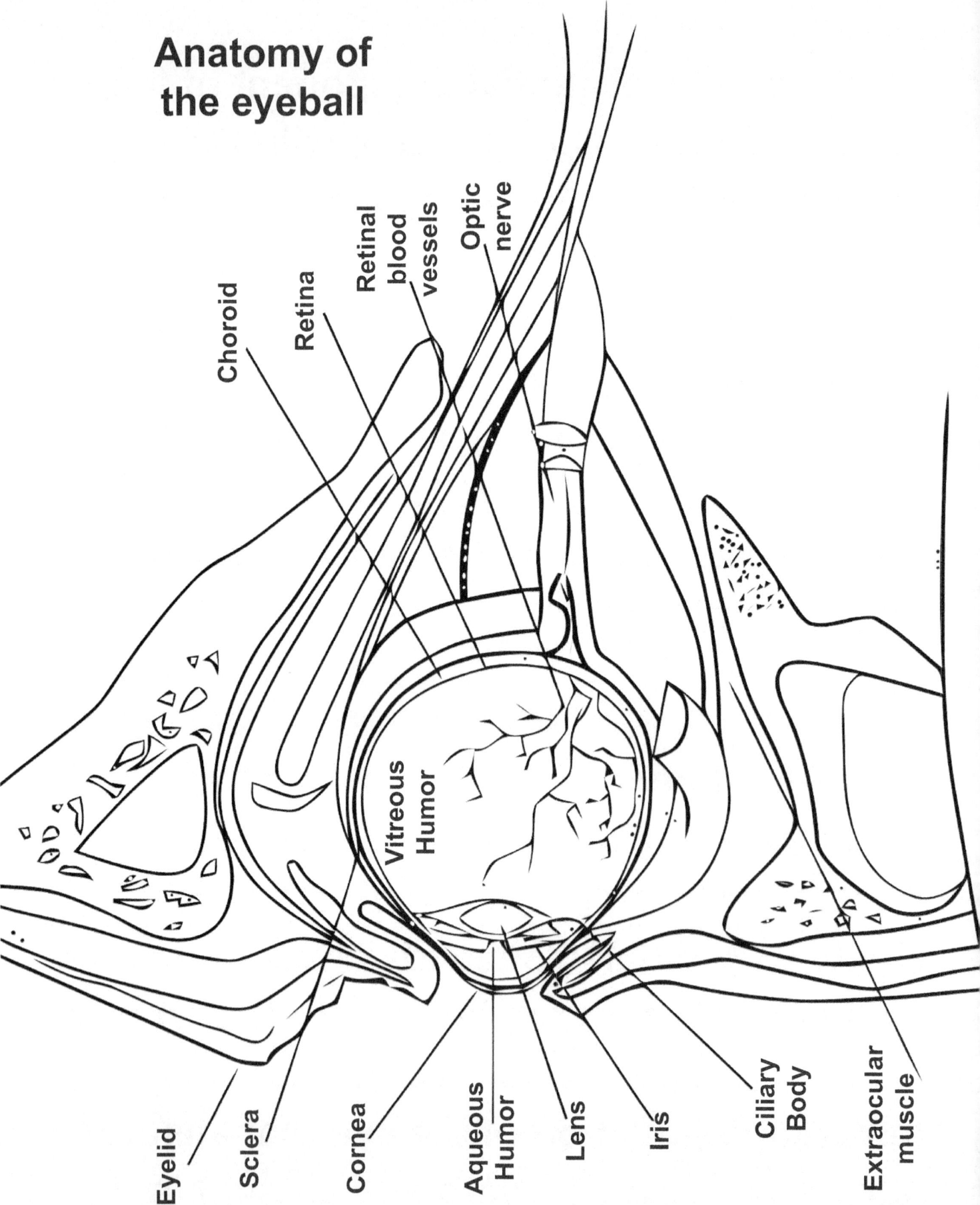

Choroid

Retina

Retinal blood vessels

Optic nerve

Vitreous Humor

Eyelid

Sclera

Cornea

Aqueous Humor

Lens

Iris

Ciliary Body

Extraocular muscle

12

The retina, situated at the posterior of the eye, consists of a delicate layer of tissue housing numerous light-sensitive cells known as photoreceptors. These remarkable cells have the ability to convert light into neural signals that can be interpreted by the brain.

Within the retina, there are two primary types of photoreceptors: rods and cones. Rods excel at detecting low levels of light and play a crucial role in night vision, while cones are responsible for capturing color information and operate optimally under bright lighting conditions. Once these cells generate signals, they are transmitted through the optic nerve towards the visual cortex where further processing takes place.

Anatomy of the eyeball

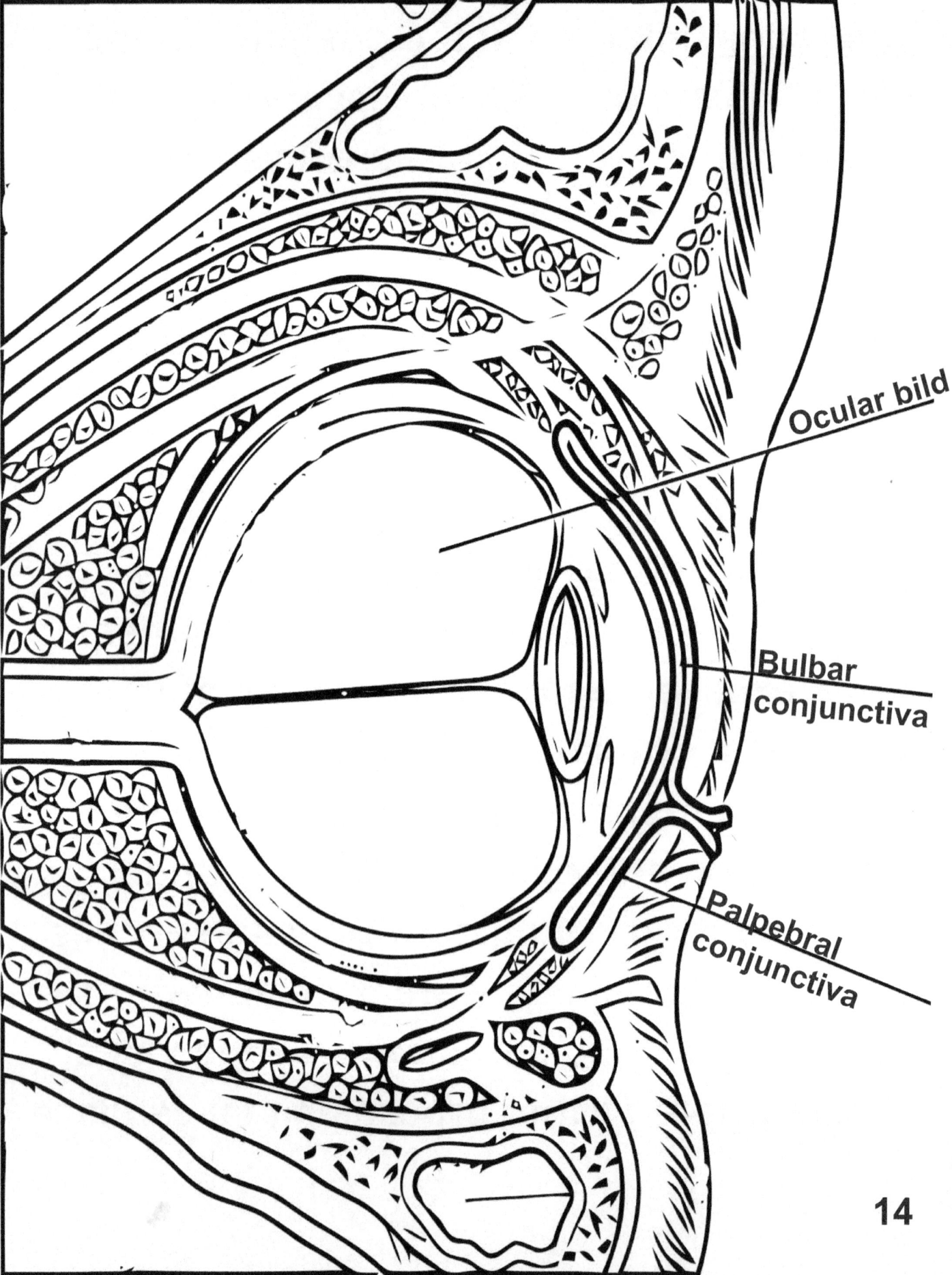

Ocular bild

Bulbar conjunctiva

Palpebral conjunctiva

14

Eye movement

The complexity and fascination of eye movement muscles are evident in their anatomy. In each eye, there are six intricate muscles that collaborate to enable us to move our eyes in all directions. These muscles attach to the eyeball and exert force from various angles, granting us the ability to gaze upward, downward, leftward, rightward, and diagonally.

The superior rectus, inferior rectus, medial rectus, lateral rectus, superior oblique, and inferior oblique constitute the six essential muscles responsible for eye movement. The superior rectus aids in elevating the eye, while the inferior rectus facilitates descent. The medial rectus moves the eye towards the nose for inward navigation while the lateral rectus accomplishes outward movements. Additionally, the superior oblique rotates the eye downwards and away from the nose while the inferior oblique assumes responsibility for upward rotation away from this central point.

Eye mouvement muscles

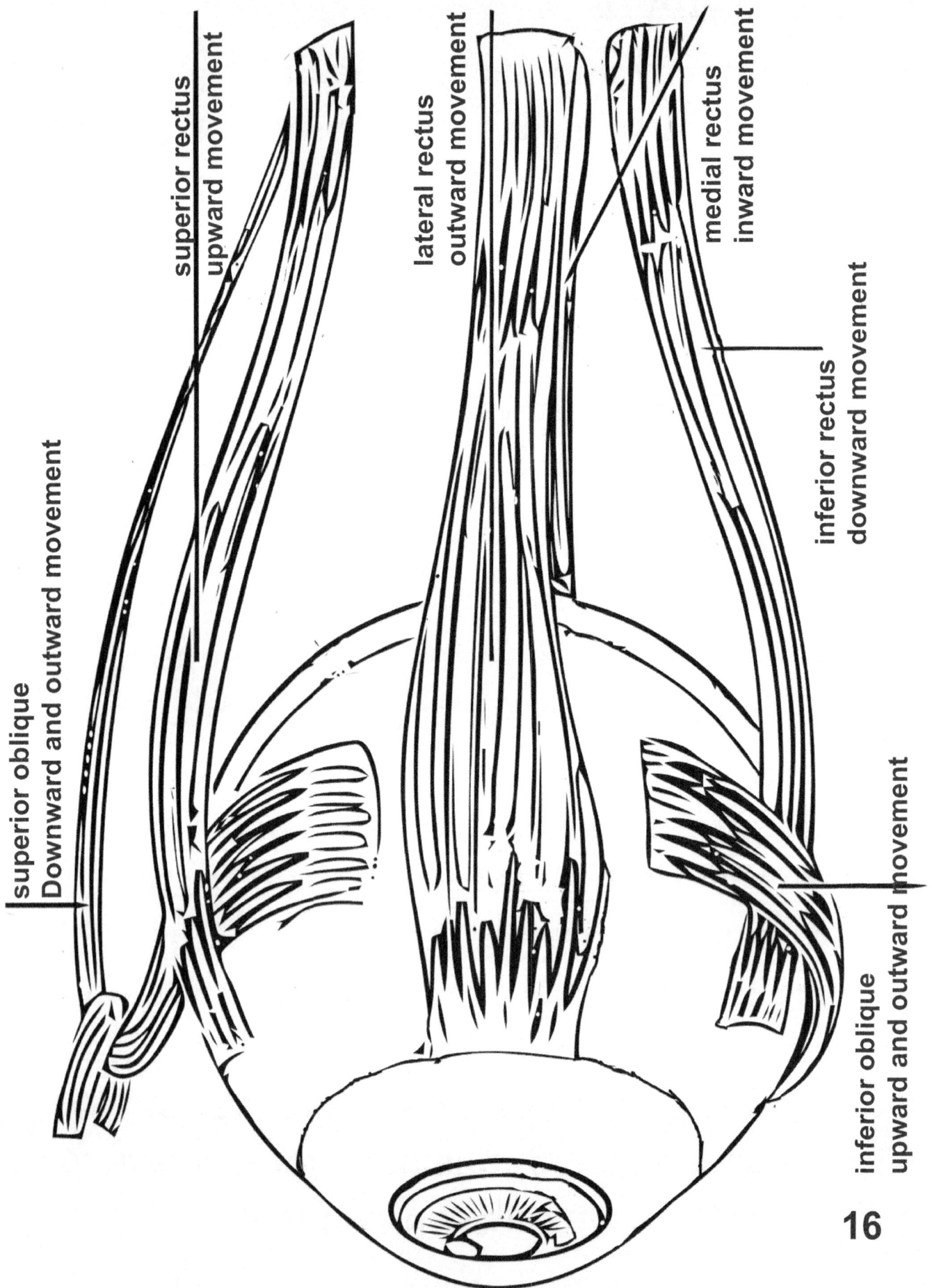

superior rectus
upward movement

lateral rectus
outward movement

medial rectus
inward movement

superior oblique
Downward and outward movement

inferior rectus
downward movement

inferior oblique
upward and outward movement

16

The intricate coordination of six different eye muscles allows us to effortlessly move our eyes and track objects. These muscles are controlled by three cranial nerves, which send signals to each muscle to execute precise movements in various directions.

For instance, when we shift our gaze to the right, the lateral rectus muscle on the right eye contracts alongside the medial rectus muscle on the left eye. This synchronized action enables both eyes to focus on a single point. Likewise, when we look upwards, the superior rectus muscles engage while the inferior oblique muscles relax, facilitating upward eye movement.

Strabismus is a prevalent eye movement disorder that affects the alignment of the eyes. If left untreated, it can lead to double vision, reduced depth perception, and potential blindness in one eye. The causes of strabismus can vary and may include genetic factors, muscle weakness, or nerve damage.

Nystagmus is another common eye movement disorder characterized by involuntary movements of the eyes. This condition can make reading, driving, and other daily activities challenging. Nystagmus can be present from birth (congenital) or develop later in life due to neurological conditions or trauma.

Strabismus

Normal vision

Binocular squint

Binocular divergent strabismus

Monocular squint

Divergent strabismus Monocular

19

The process of diagnosing eye movement disorders can be quite complex and involves a range of tests. One commonly used test is the cover test, which requires the patient to focus on an object while the doctor covers one eye at a time. This examination helps to identify any misalignment or deviation in the eyes. Additional tests may include assessing the range of motion in the eyes or using specialized equipment to track eye movements.

Treatment options for eye movement disorders vary depending on the specific disorder and its severity. In some cases, wearing corrective lenses or engaging in targeted eye exercises may be sufficient to alleviate symptoms. However, more severe cases may necessitate surgical intervention to correct muscle imbalances or other underlying issues.

Strabismus surgery

After

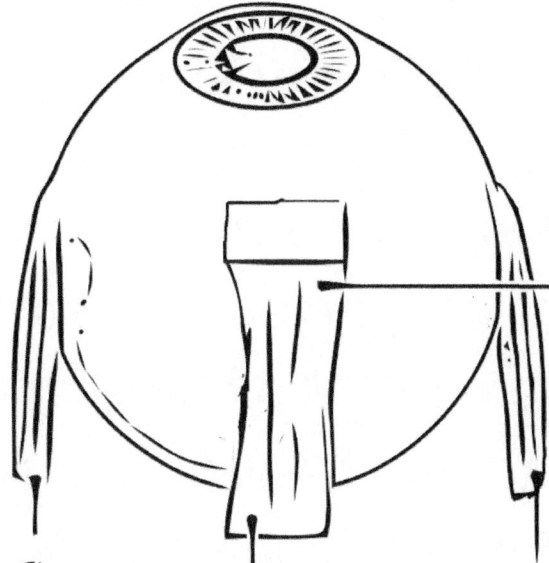

New Position

Superior rectus muscle

Lateral rectus muscle

Inferior rectus muscle

Before

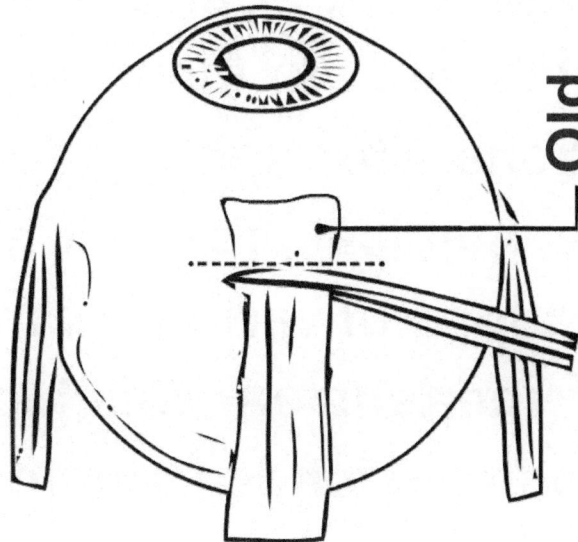

Old Position

21

The human retina is an incredibly fascinating part of our anatomy. Its primary function is to capture light and convert it into electrical signals that are then sent to the brain, enabling us to perceive and comprehend the world around us. The absence of the retina would deprive us of the ability to witness the breathtaking beauty of a sunrise or experience pure delight in seeing a loved one's radiant smile.

Despite its relatively small size, the retina holds immense significance in our visual system. It has often been metaphorically described as a 'window to the soul' due to its ability to provide insights into our innermost thoughts and emotions. Through careful examination of the retina, medical professionals can identify indications of various ailments such as diabetes and hypertension. This highlights that the role of the retina extends beyond just vision; it actively contributes to our overall health and well-being.

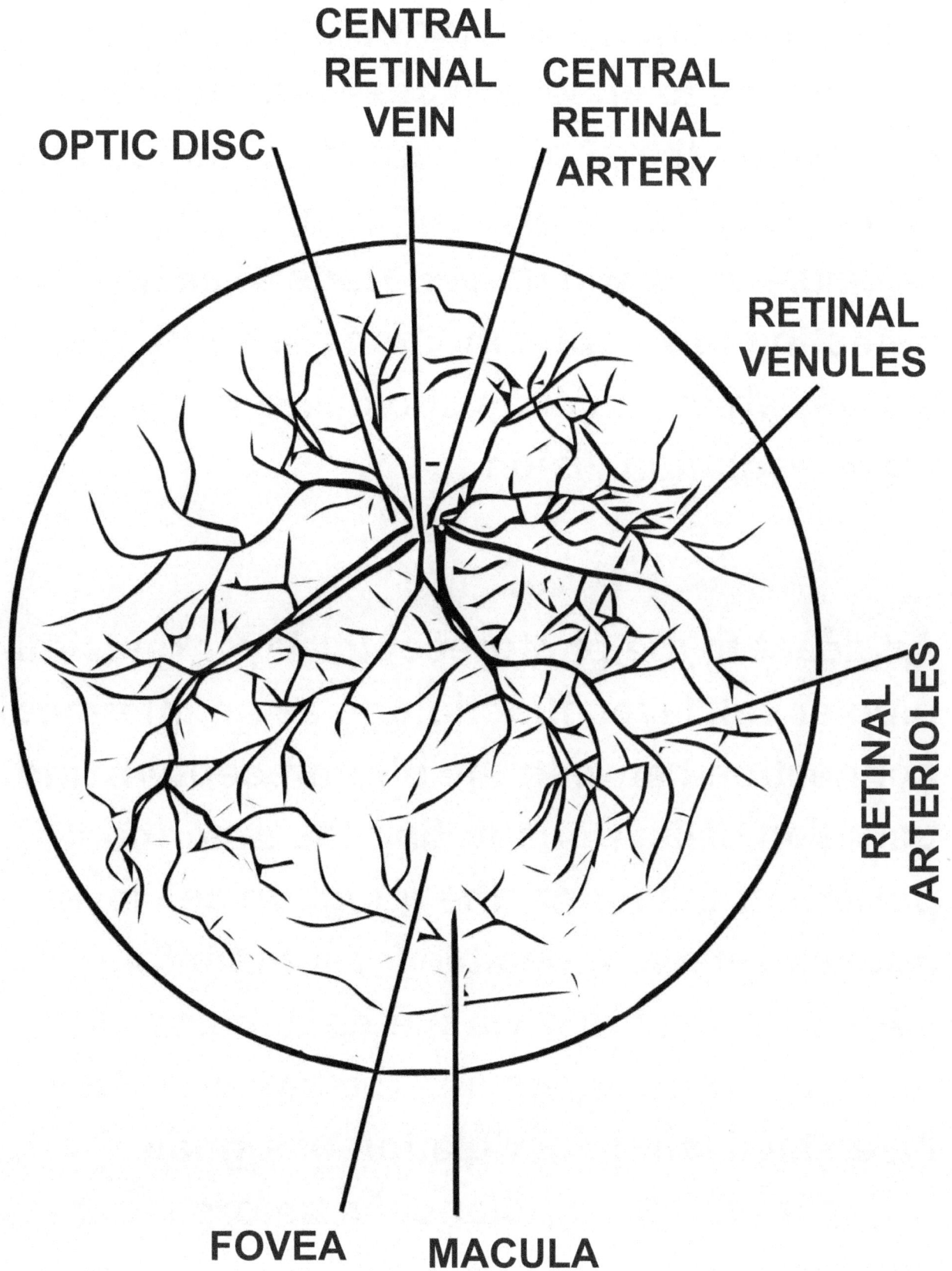

THE RETINA

CENTRAL
RETINAL
VEIN

CENTRAL
RETINAL
ARTERY

OPTIC DISC

RETINAL
VENULES

RETINAL
ARTERIOLES

FOVEA

MACULA

The retina is a highly intricate structure with distinct layers, each playing a vital role. The pigmented epithelium forms the outermost layer and serves to absorb excess light while nourishing the photoreceptors. Situated beneath is the photoreceptor layer comprising two types of cells—rods and cones. Rods excel in detecting low-light conditions essential for night vision, whereas cones specialize in color and high-resolution vision.

Adjacent to the photoreceptor layer rests the bipolar cell layer, functioning as an intermediate connection between the photoreceptors and ganglion cells. Constituting the innermost portion of the retina, the ganglion cell layer houses cells responsible for transmitting signals to the brain via the optic nerve. Resting between these layers lies the amacrine cell layer, facilitating modulation of signals originating from bipolar cells before reaching ganglion cells.

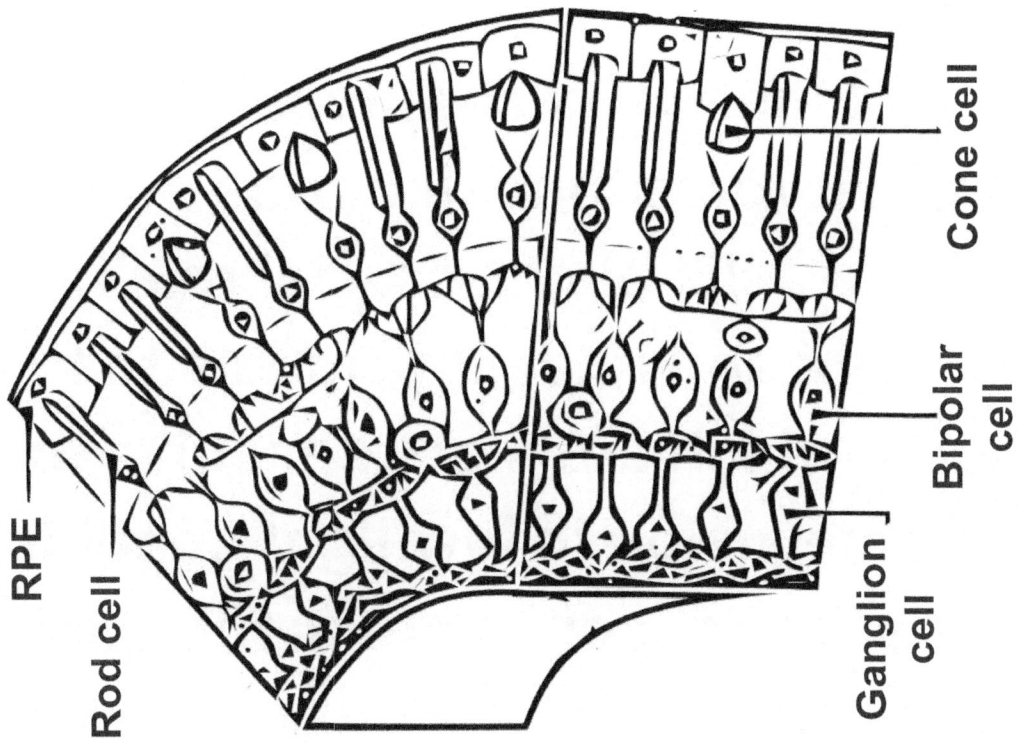

RPE

Rod cell

Cone cell

Bipolar cell

Ganglion cell

Section of Retina

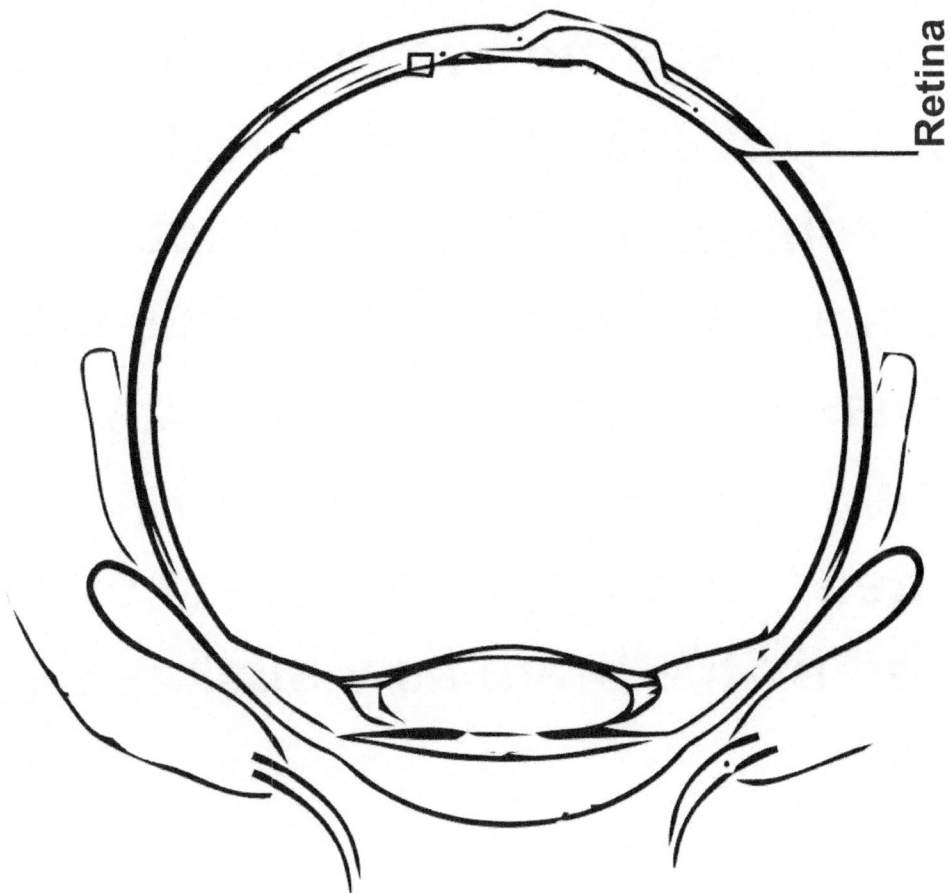

Retina

The retina of the eye is composed of two types of photoreceptor cells: rods and cones. These cells play a crucial role in detecting light and relaying signals to the brain. Rods, which are more sensitive to light, facilitate vision in low-light conditions. On the other hand, cones are responsible for color vision and enhancing sharpness and detail in bright light.

When light enters the eye, it interacts with the photopigments present in rods and cones, leading to a chemical reaction that generates an electrical signal. This signal then travels through a complex network of cells within the retina before being transmitted to the optic nerve and eventually processed by the brain as visual information.

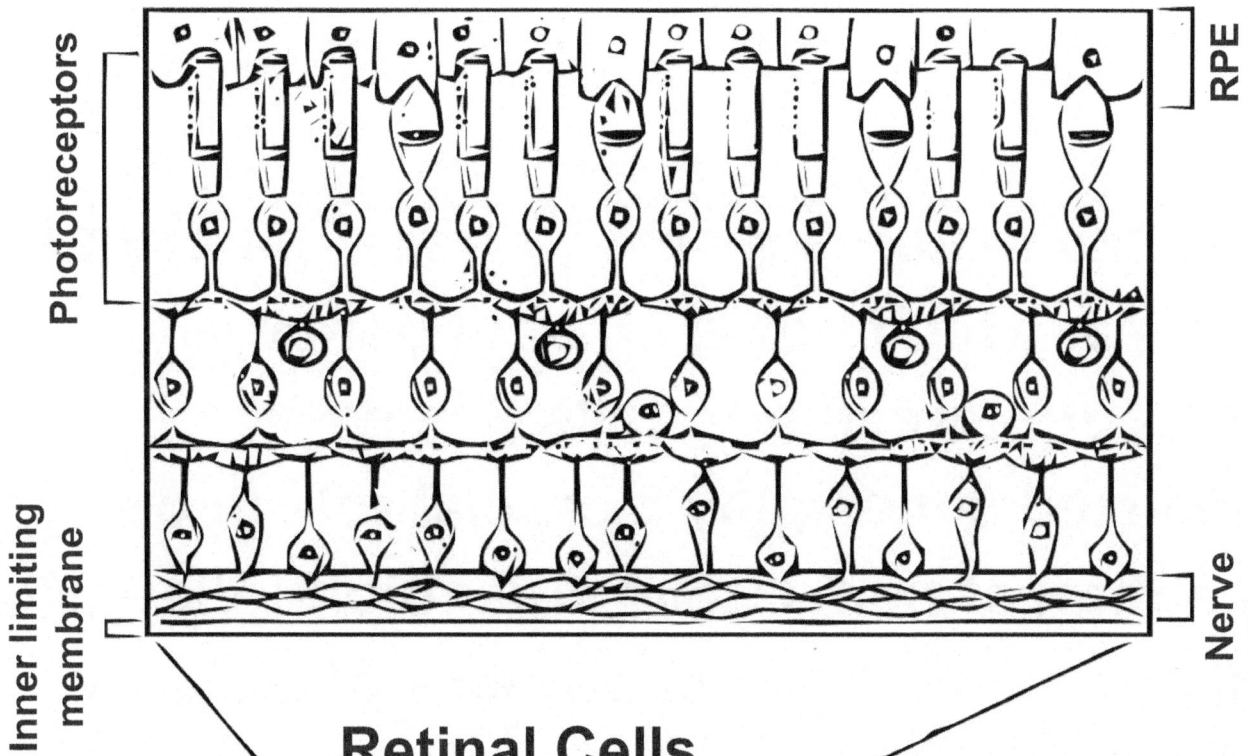

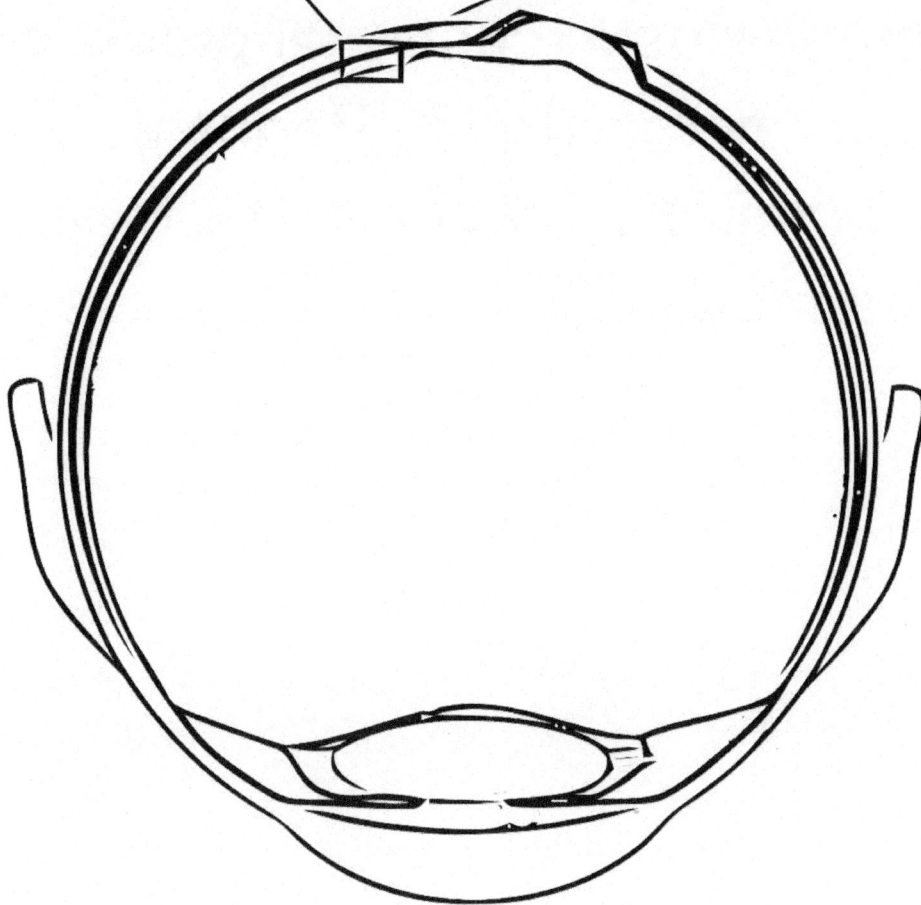

Retinal Cells

RPE

Photoreceptors

Inner limiting membrane

Nerve fiber

Rod Cell

Cone Cell

Ganglion Cell

Bipolar Cell

Amacrine Cell

Horizontal Cell

27

The retina features a small, central pit called the fovea, which holds an abundance of cones - photoreceptor cells. These specialized cones play a crucial role in our perception of fine details and colors. Visual acuity pertains to the sharpness and clarity of our vision. When we gaze directly at an object, the light from said object aligns with the fovea, granting us exceptional precision and clearness in perceiving it. Hence why the fovea is commonly known as the focal point of our attention.

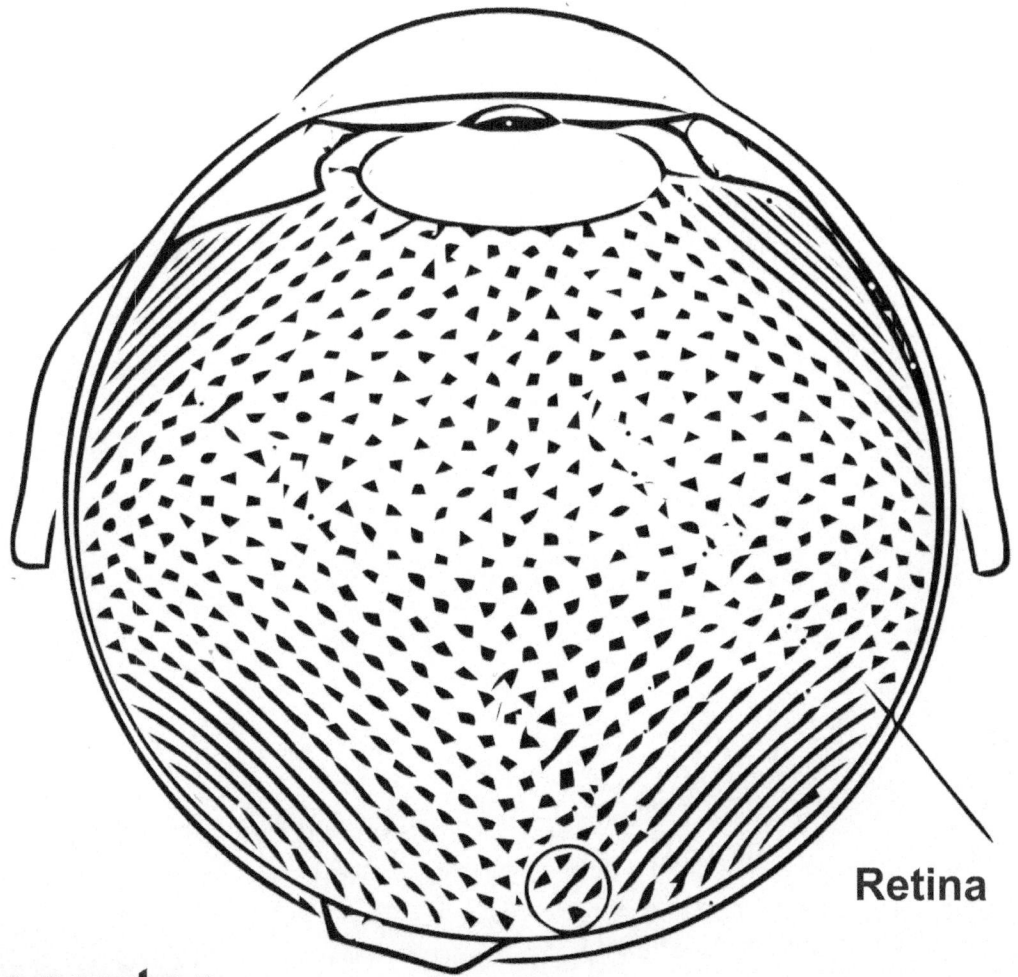

Retina

Photoreceptor cells

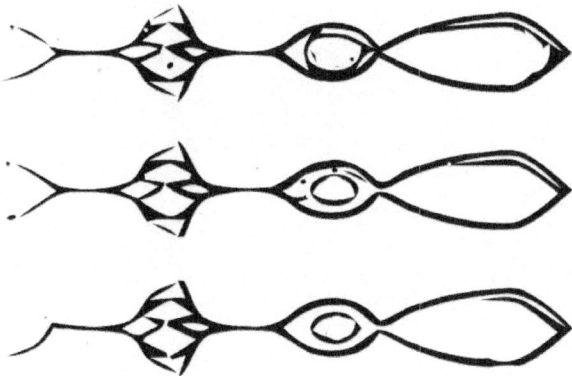

Cone Cell

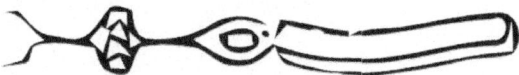

Rod Cell

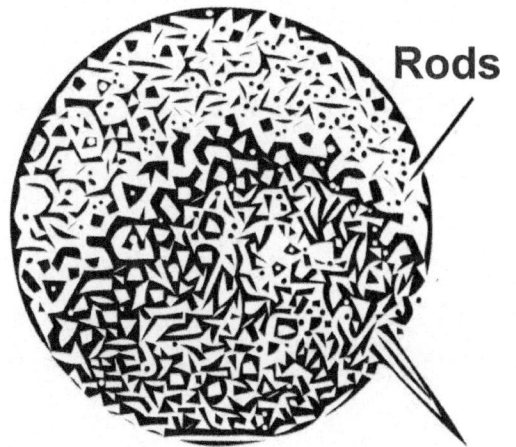

Rods

Cones

29

Photoreceptor cells

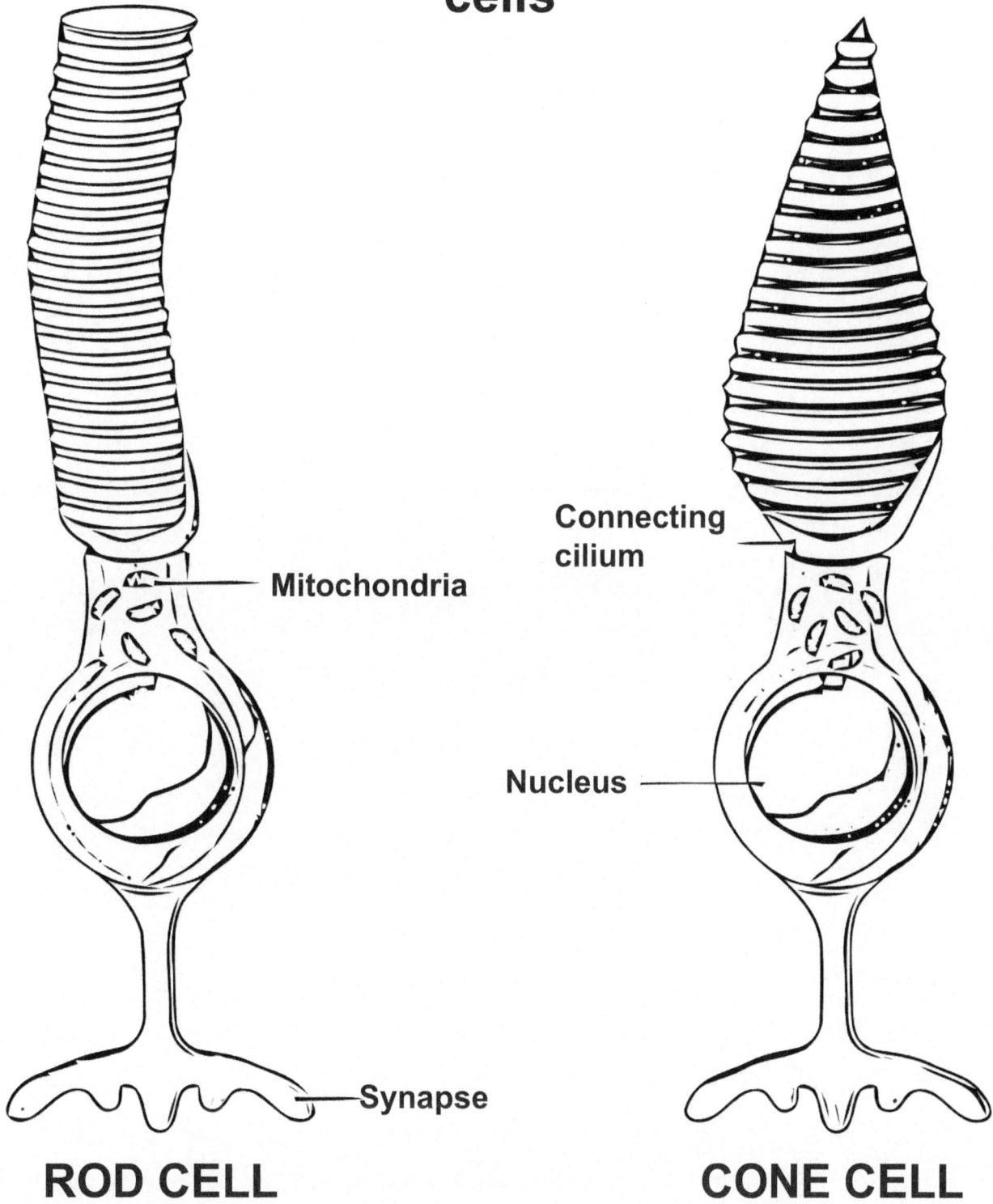

Mitochondria

Connecting cilium

Nucleus

Synapse

ROD CELL

CONE CELL

Retinopathy

Macular degeneration is a prevalent condition that leads to the deterioration of vision in individuals over 50 years old. It specifically affects the macula, which is responsible for providing clear and central vision. Dry macular degeneration progresses gradually, whereas wet macular degeneration can result in rapid and severe vision impairment.

Diabetic retinopathy is a complication of diabetes that impacts the blood vessels within the retina. If left untreated, it can cause loss of vision or even blindness. Individuals with diabetes are at a heightened risk of developing this condition, particularly if their blood sugar levels are poorly managed.

Retinal detachment occurs when the retina becomes detached from its underlying tissue. Failure to promptly undergo treatment can lead to significant vision loss or complete blindness. Risk factors for retinal detachment include nearsightedness, previous eye injuries or surgeries, as well as having a family history of this condition.

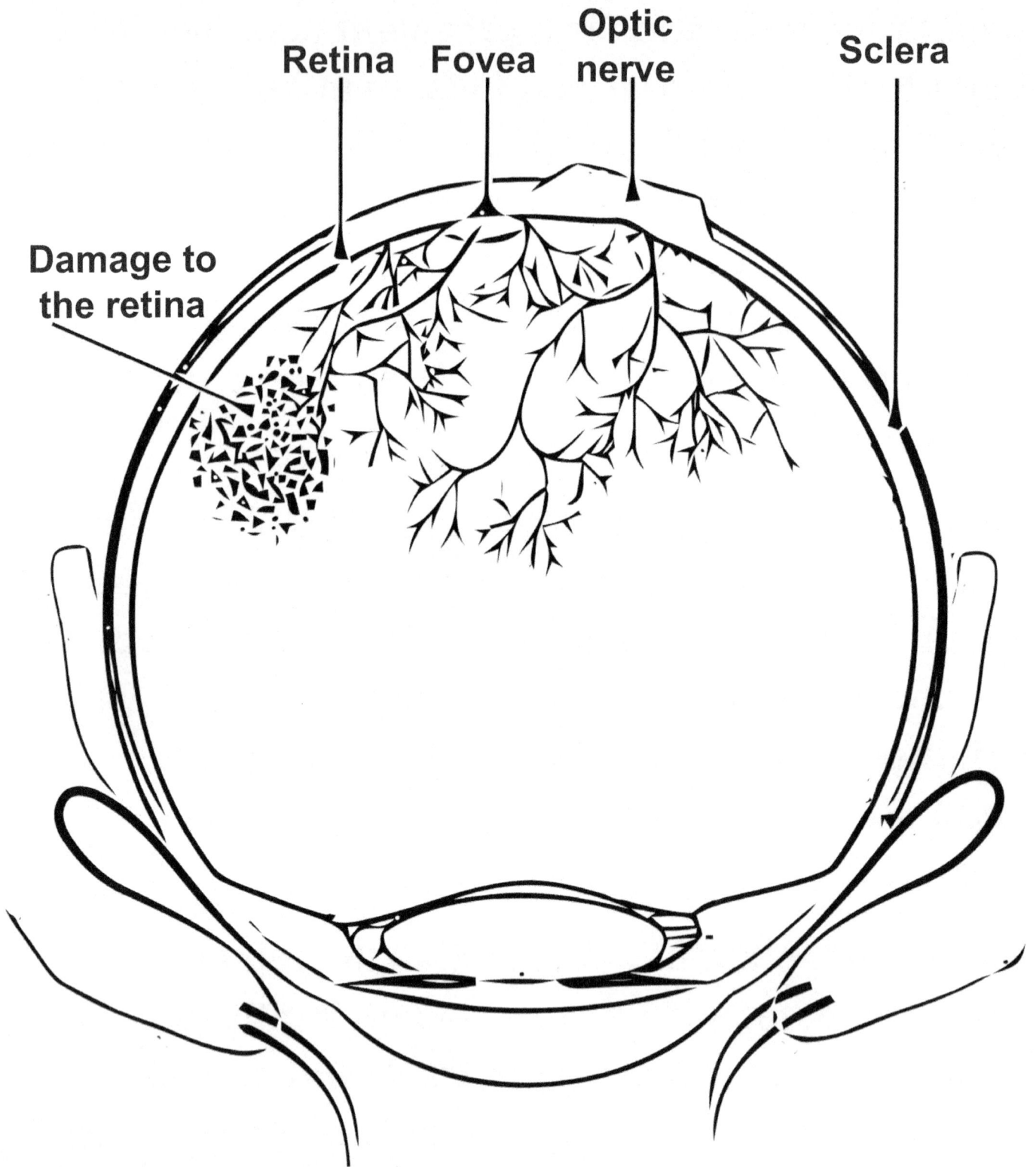

Retina   Fovea   Optic nerve   Sclera

Damage to the retina

Retinopathy

Macular degeneration is a complex disease that affects the macula, an essential part of the eye responsible for central vision. There are two primary forms of macular degeneration: dry and wet.

Dry macular degeneration is the more prevalent type and progresses slowly over time. It occurs when the macula thins out and accumulates small yellow deposits known as drusen. Conversely, wet macular degeneration is less common but more severe. It arises from the growth of abnormal blood vessels beneath the macula, leading to fluid leakage and damage to this vital area.

To convey these distinctions effectively, visual aids such as diagrams and charts can be employed to better illustrate the disparities between dry and wet macular degeneration. For instance, an image could portray the thinning of the macula in dry macular degeneration alongside the abnormal blood vessel growth in its wet counterpart. Furthermore, real-life examples such as difficulties with reading or recognizing faces can be highlighted to help audiences comprehend the impact associated with each variant of this condition.

Macular degeneration presents itself in various forms, with several prevalent symptoms. Individuals may experience blurred or hazy vision, challenges in reading and recognizing faces, and distorted vision that causes straight lines to appear wavy or crooked.

Another indicator of macular degeneration is the emergence of blind spots or dark patches in the center of one's visual field. Such impediments can make carrying out everyday activities such as driving or cooking challenging and can significantly affect one's overall quality of life.

The biggest risk factor for macular degeneration is age, with a higher occurrence rate in individuals over the age of 60. Genetics also play a significant role, as those with a family history of the disease are more susceptible to developing it. Lifestyle choices, such as smoking, an unhealthy diet, and lack of physical activity, can further increase the likelihood of macular degeneration.

Detecting and preventing macular degeneration early on is crucial for effective management. Regular eye exams play a vital role in identifying the disease in its initial stages, offering patients a greater chance at successful treatment. Adopting healthy lifestyle habits like quitting smoking and consuming a nutritious diet filled with fruits and vegetables can also help decrease the risk of developing macular degeneration.

Treatment

There are multiple treatment options available for individuals with macular degeneration, including medication, laser therapy, and surgery. Each option has its own advantages and disadvantages, making it crucial to consult with a healthcare professional to determine the most suitable treatment for your specific condition.

Medications can be beneficial in slowing down the progression of macular degeneration and reducing the risk of vision loss. However, it's important to note that they may come with potential side effects and require regular injections or monitoring.

Laser therapy is another treatment option that aims to seal leaking blood vessels in the eye and prevent further damage. It's worth mentioning that this approach may not be effective for everyone and could cause some discomfort during the procedure.

Macular Degeneration

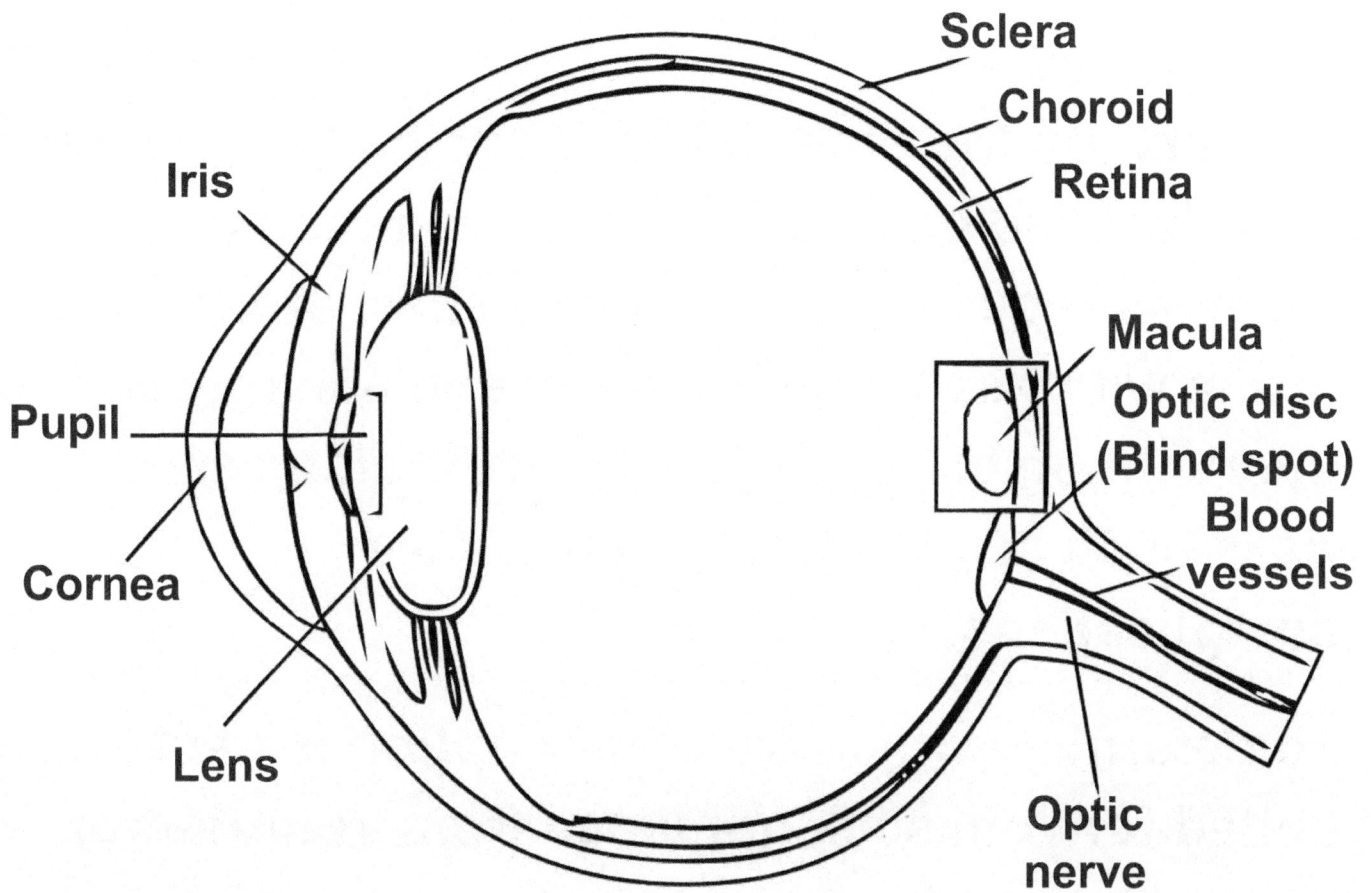

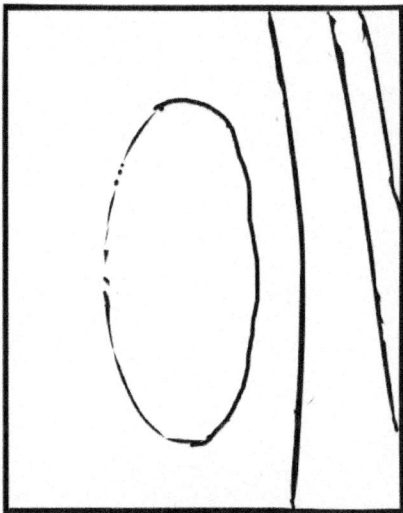

Sclera
Choroid
Retina

Iris

Macula
Optic disc
(Blind spot)
Blood
vessels

Pupil

Cornea

Lens

Optic
nerve

Normal

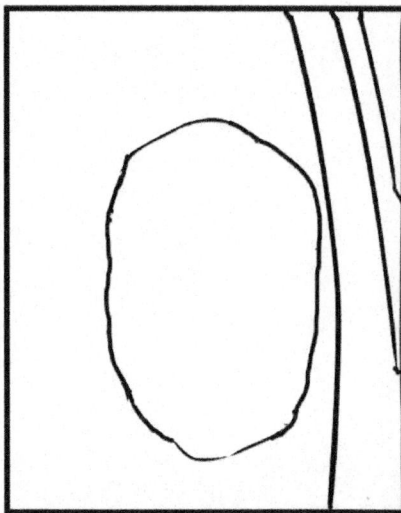

'Wet' macular
degeneration

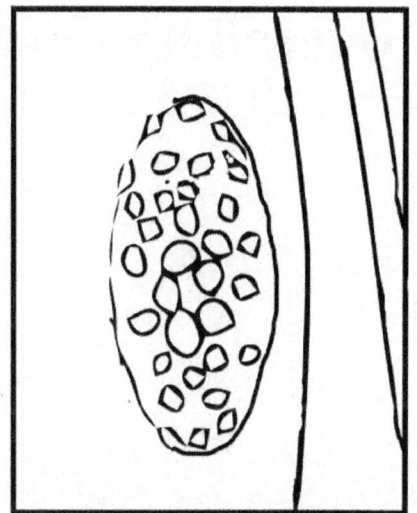

'Dry' macular
degeneration

Surgery, on the other hand, is typically reserved for advanced cases of macular degeneration. It involves replacing the damaged part of the retina with healthy tissue. While this surgical intervention can improve vision, it also carries risks such as infection and possible complications.

To determine which treatment option is best suited for you, seek guidance from your doctor who will consider various factors such as the stage of your macular degeneration and your overall health.

Wet Macular Degeneration

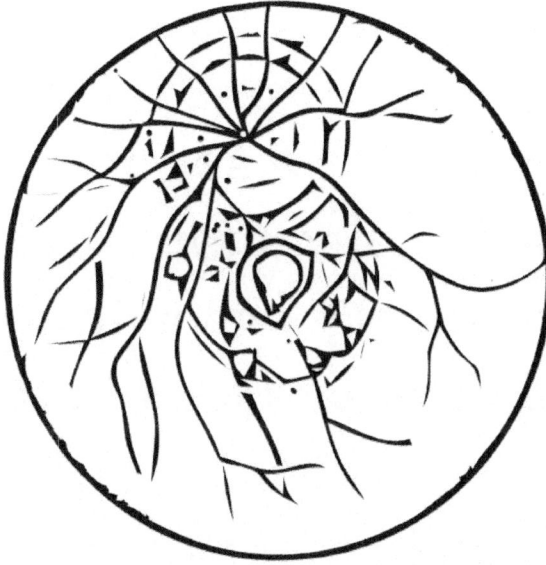

Blind spot in center of the vision

Dry Macular Degeneration

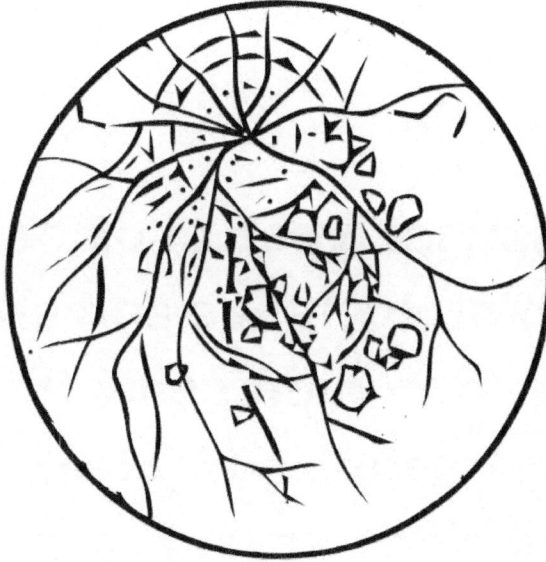

Unusually fuzzy or distorted vision

Normal Eye

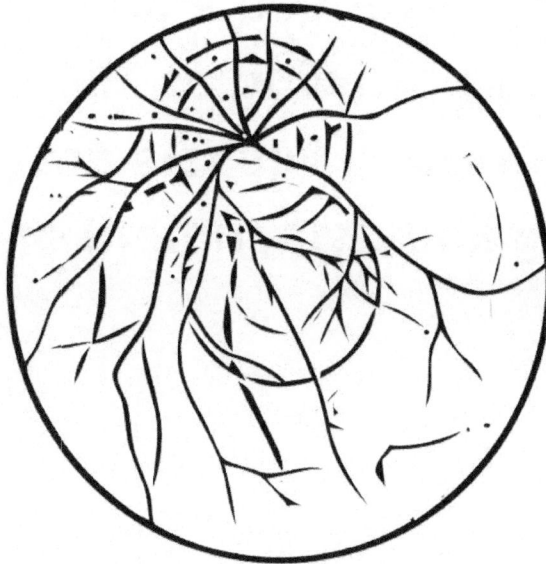

Clear vision of normal eyes

41

Diabetic retinopathy is a serious complication of diabetes that specifically affects the eyes. It arises as a result of chronically elevated blood sugar levels, which leads to damage of the blood vessels in the retina - the light-sensing part of the eye responsible for transmitting signals to the brain. Over time, this damage can progressively impair vision and ultimately cause blindness.

There are two distinct types of diabetic retinopathy: non-proliferative and proliferative. The non-proliferative form represents the early stage of the condition, characterized by leakage of fluid or blood from small blood vessels within the retina. Proliferative diabetic retinopathy, on the other hand, denotes an advanced stage where abnormal blood vessels start growing on the surface of the retina. These newfound vessels are prone to causing scarring and detachment of the retina itself.

The presence of diabetic retinopathy can lead to a range of symptoms that have a significant impact on an individual's daily activities. One such symptom is the occurrence of blurred vision, which poses challenges in reading, driving, and even recognizing faces. This can be especially distressing for individuals who heavily rely on their visual acuity for their profession or hobbies.

Additionally, another symptom associated with diabetic retinopathy is the appearance of floaters in one's vision. These are tiny specks or clouds that appear to drift across the field of sight. While they may not always cause discomfort, they can prove to be distracting and impede one's ability to concentrate on tasks at hand.

Furthermore, individuals with this condition often experience difficulties in seeing clearly in low-light conditions, particularly at night. This can create obstacles when attempting to navigate through poorly illuminated environments.

Controlling blood sugar levels is a highly effective method for preventing diabetic retinopathy. To achieve this, it is crucial to adopt a comprehensive approach encompassing diet, exercise, and medication. It is imperative to collaborate closely with your healthcare provider in order to devise a personalized plan that suits you best.

In addition to glucose control, regular eye examinations play a pivotal role in averting the onset of diabetic retinopathy. By detecting early indications of the condition, an eye specialist can work in tandem with you to effectively manage it before it advances further. Various treatment options are available for diabetic retinopathy, ranging from medications and laser surgery to lifestyle modifications such as smoking cessation and maintaining an optimal weight.

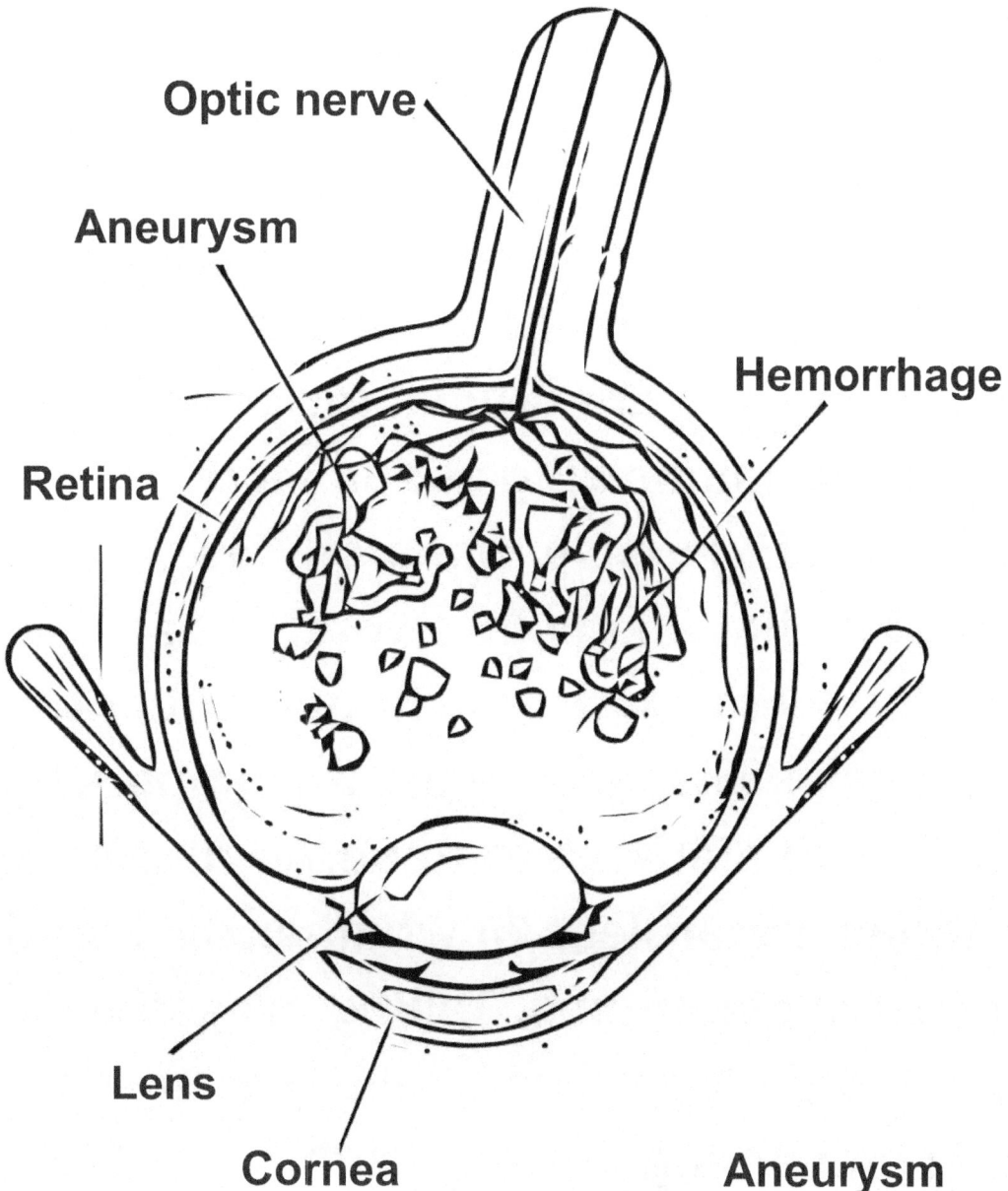

Optic nerve

Aneurysm

Hemorrhage

Retina

Lens

Cornea

Diabetic retinopathy

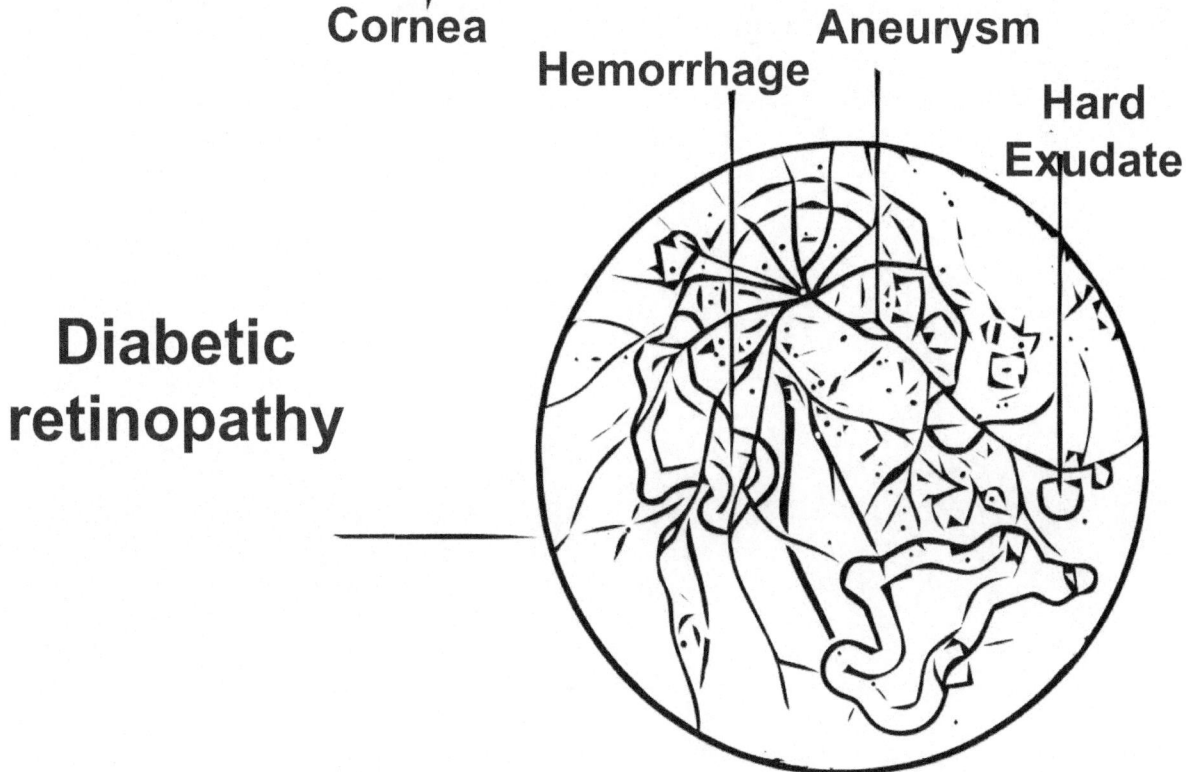

Hemorrhage

Aneurysm

Hard Exudate

The early identification and proper management of diabetic retinopathy are crucial for preventing vision loss and minimizing associated complications. Extensive research has demonstrated that timely intervention can significantly decrease the likelihood of blindness by as much as 95%. As a result, it is imperative for individuals with diabetes to undergo routine eye examinations, regardless of whether they exhibit any noticeable symptoms. Taking proactive measures in this regard can have a dramatic impact on preserving visual health.

Normal

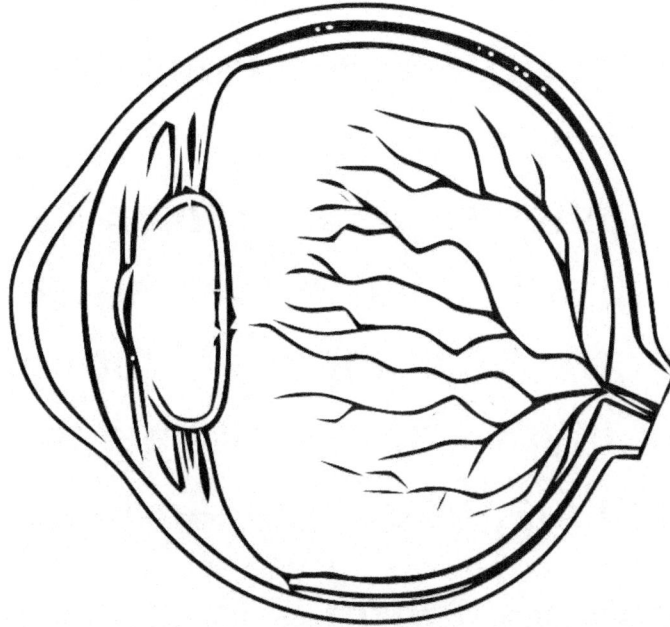

Diabetic retinopathy

Nonproliferative Retinopathy

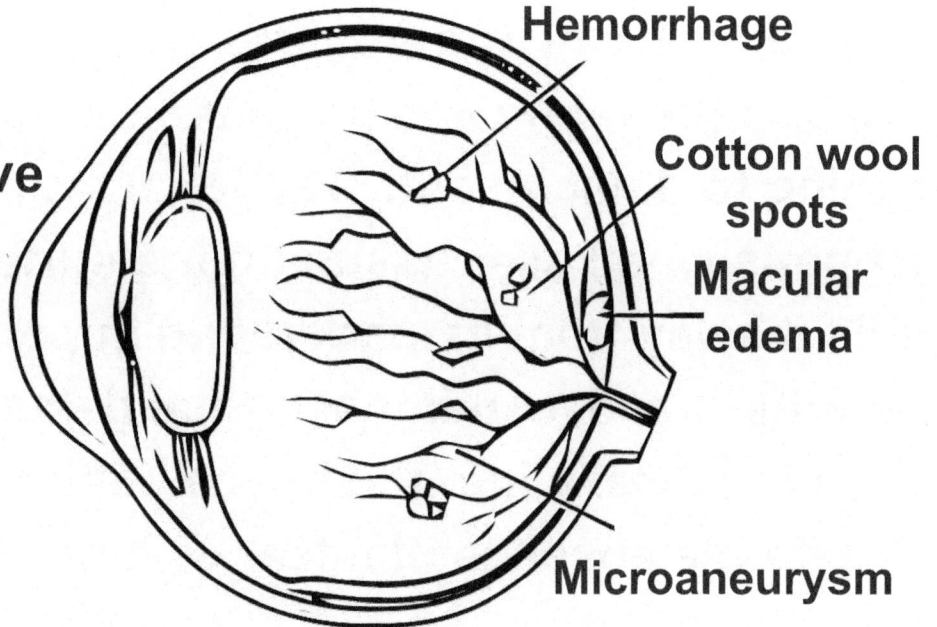

Hemorrhage

Cotton wool spots

Macular edema

Microaneurysm

Proliferative Retinopathy

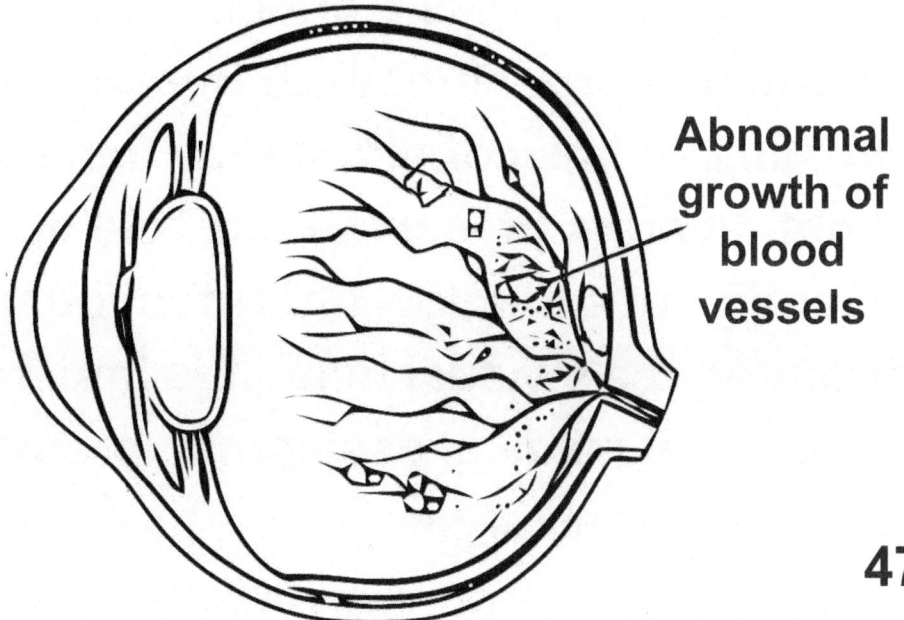

Abnormal growth of blood vessels

47

Retinal detachment is a critical condition that arises when the retina, a delicate layer of tissue at the rear of the eye, becomes separated from its underlying supportive tissue. If left untreated, this can result in vision loss or even complete blindness. There are three distinct types of retinal detachment: rhegmatogenous, tractional, and exudative.

The most prevalent form is rhegmatogenous retinal detachment, which transpires when a tear or hole forms in the retina and permits fluid to seep through, leading to detachment. Tractional retinal detachment happens when scar tissue on the surface of the retina pulls it away from its underlying support tissue. On the other hand, exudative retinal detachment occurs when fluid leaks into the space behind the retina despite the absence of a tear or hole.

Retinal detachment is a critical condition that necessitates urgent medical intervention. Common indicators of this condition may include abrupt flashes of light, floaters present in the field of vision, or the perception of a shadow or curtain obstructing a portion of one's visual field. It is imperative to seek professional medical assistance promptly if any of these symptoms arise.

There are various factors that can contribute to the occurrence of retinal detachment, including trauma, aging, and underlying medical conditions. In cases where the eye experiences trauma, such as a blow or injury, the retina can detach from the back of the eye. As we age, the vitreous gel inside our eyes begins to shrink and pull away from the retina, increasing the risk of retinal detachment. Additionally, certain medical conditions like diabetes and nearsightedness can also elevate the likelihood of this condition.

Other underlying medical issues such as sickle cell disease, tumors, and inflammatory disorders can also lead to retinal detachment. It is important to keep in mind that retinal detachment may sometimes occur without any apparent cause. Furthermore, genetic factors may play a role in its development.

It is imperative to seek immediate medical attention for retinal detachment, a grave condition. Thankfully, there are numerous effective treatment options available to restore vision and prevent further damage to the retina.

Surgery stands as the most common method for treating retinal detachment. During this procedure, a skilled surgeon will reattach the retina using small stitches or a specialized laser. The choice of surgery depends on the severity and location of the detachment. In certain instances, a gas bubble may be injected into the eye to facilitate holding the retina in place during the healing process. Additionally, laser therapy can be applied to seal any tears or holes in the retina and halt subsequent detachment.

Retinal detachment

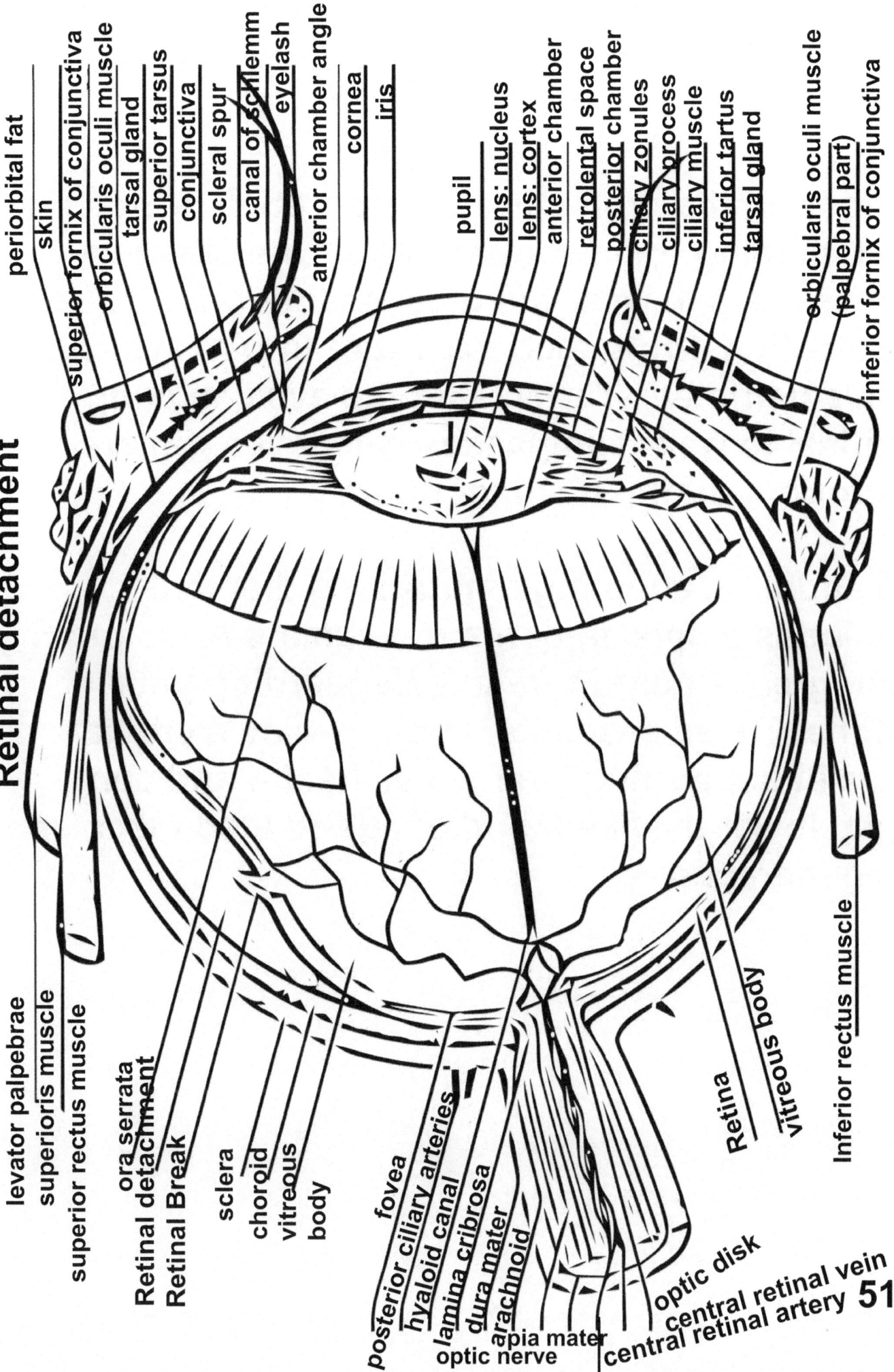

periorbital fat

skin

superior fornix of conjunctiva

orbicularis oculi muscle

tarsal gland

superior tarsus

conjunctiva

scleral spur

canal of Schlemm

eyelash

anterior chamber angle

cornea

iris

pupil

lens: nucleus

lens: cortex

anterior chamber

retrolental space

posterior chamber

ciliary zonules

ciliary process

ciliary muscle

inferior tartus

tarsal gland

orbicularis oculi muscle (palpebral part)

inferior fornix of conjunctiva

levator palpebrae superioris muscle

superior rectus muscle

ora serrata

Retinal detachment

Retinal Break

sclera

choroid

vitreous body

fovea

posterior ciliary arteries

hyaloid canal

lamina cribrosa

dura mater

arachnoid

apia mater

optic nerve

Retina

vitreous body

Inferior rectus muscle

optic disk

central retinal vein

central retinal artery 51

Ensuring the protection of your retina is vital for maintaining optimal eye health. One effective measure is to wear sunglasses that offer UV ray protection. Prolonged exposure to UV rays can have detrimental effects on the eyes, making it critical to wear sunglasses whenever you are outdoors during daylight hours.

In addition, adopting a nutritious diet that includes ample amounts of vitamins A, C, and E can greatly contribute to safeguarding your retina. These essential vitamins play a crucial role in supporting overall eye health and can help lower the likelihood of age-related macular degeneration.

Visual System

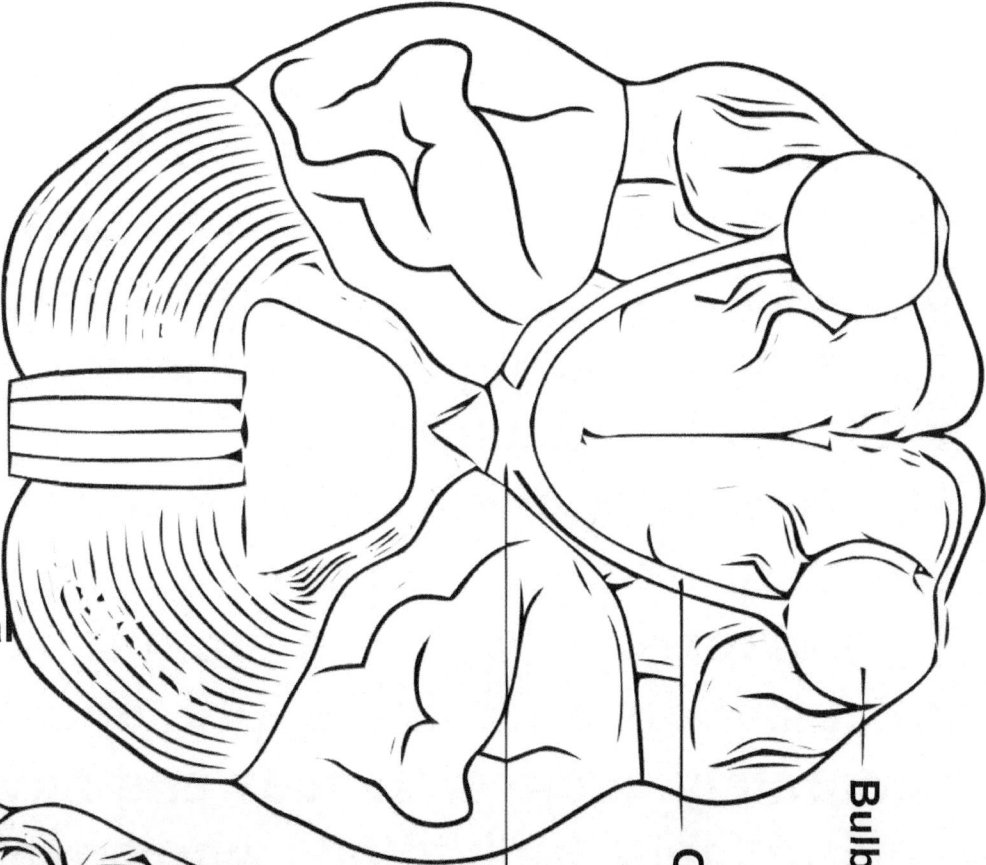

Primary visual cortex

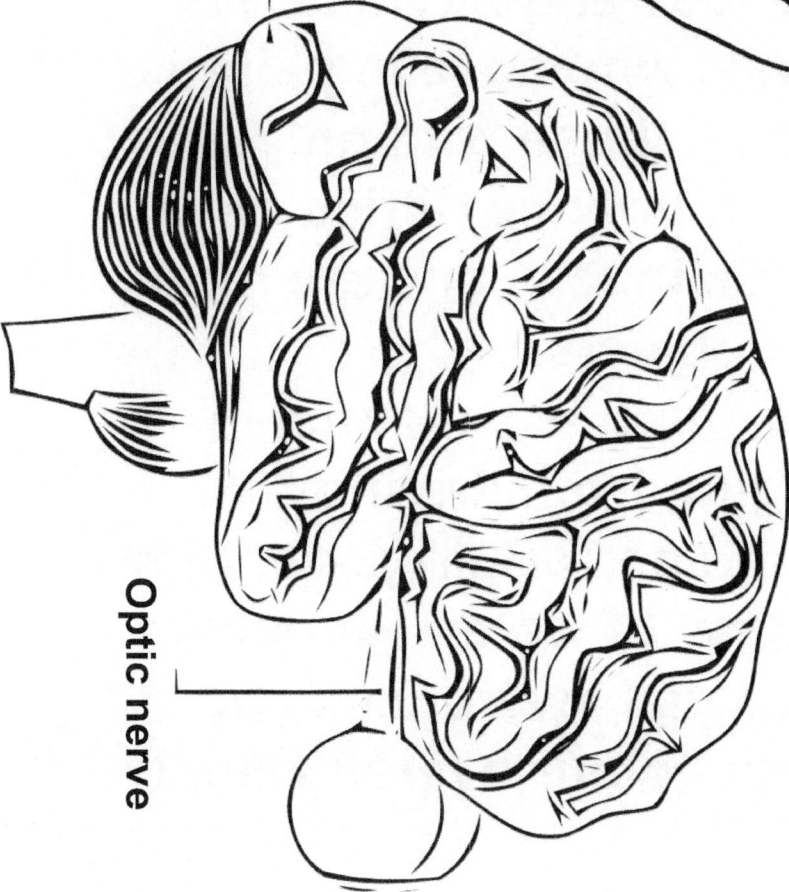

Optic nerve

Optic Chiasm

Optic nerve

Bulb of eye

Binocular vision

The binocular vision system plays a vital role in our ability to perceive the world around us in three dimensions. Through a sophisticated process, our eyes work together as a team, combining information to create a single image with depth and dimension.

One key component of binocular vision is the slight variation in perspective between each eye. This disparity allows the brain to accurately calculate distance and depth, enabling us to accurately judge distances and navigate our environment. Individuals who have impaired binocular vision, such as those with only one functioning eye, may experience difficulty in accurately perceiving distances and are more prone to collision with objects.

The ability to perceive depth is essential for various activities, ranging from driving and participating in sports to performing everyday tasks like pouring a glass of water. Binocular vision enhances our spatial awareness and contributes significantly to our overall visual perception.

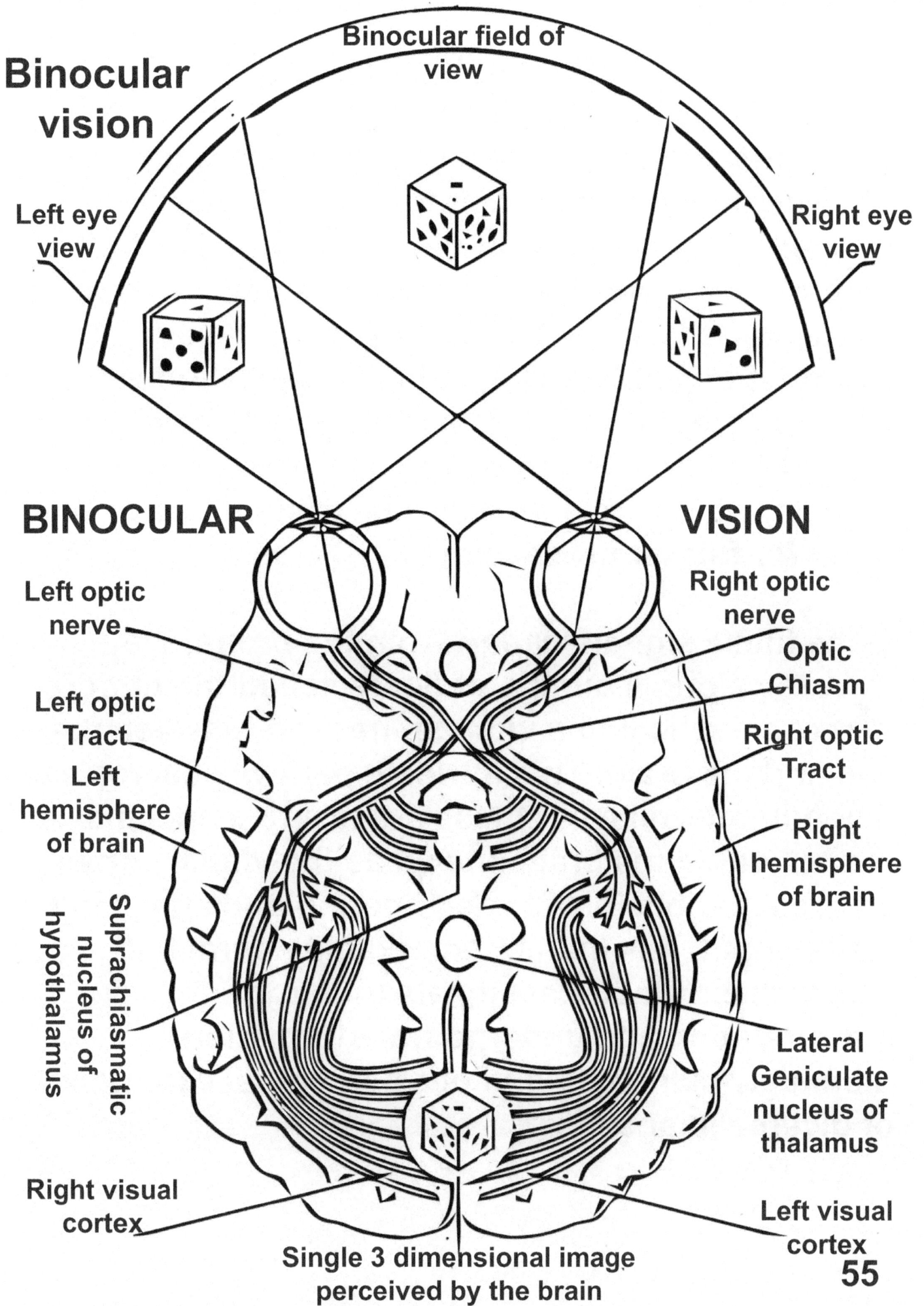

Binocular vision

Binocular field of view

Left eye view

Right eye view

BINOCULAR

VISION

Left optic nerve

Right optic nerve

Optic Chiasm

Left optic Tract

Right optic Tract

Left hemisphere of brain

Right hemisphere of brain

Suprachiasmatic nucleus of hypothalamus

Lateral Geniculate nucleus of thalamus

Right visual cortex

Left visual cortex

Single 3 dimensional image perceived by the brain

Visual Pathways

The visual pathways are a highly intricate network of structures that collaborate to enable our perception of the surrounding environment. At the core of this system lies the retina, a delicate layer of tissue located at the posterior part of the eye, comprising millions of specialized cells known as photoreceptors. These remarkable cells have the crucial function of converting light into electrical signals, which are subsequently transmitted to the brain for further processing.

Once these signals depart from the retina, they traverse along a bundle of fibers called the optic nerve, establishing a vital connection between the eye and the brain. This intricate pathway serves as a conduit for relaying these signals to a specific region within the brain known as the visual cortex - an area responsible for deciphering and analyzing visual input. It is in this remarkable neural hub where these electrical signals undergo interpretation and undergo transformation, ultimately culminating in our perceptual experience of diverse images.

Visual pathways play a crucial role in the processing of visual information, as they are responsible for transmitting this information from the eyes to the brain. Within these pathways, various types of cells work together to ensure the seamless transmission of visual data. This includes photoreceptor cells found in the retina, ganglion cells located in the optic nerve, and specialized neurons within the visual cortex.

The journey of visual information begins with light entering the eye and triggering a response in photoreceptor cells within the retina. These remarkable cells then transmit signals to bipolar cells, which subsequently activate ganglion cells. The axons of these ganglion cells converge to form what we know as the optic nerve, which serves as a conduit for transmitting visual information directly to the brain.

Once inside the brain, this incoming visual data is meticulously processed by an intricate network of neurons within the visual cortex. It is through this sophisticated process that we are able to perceive and make sense of our surrounding environment.

In summary, visual pathways serve as an essential link between our eyes and our ability to see and comprehend our surroundings. Through their complex interactions, these pathways enable us to experience and interpret the world around us with unparalleled clarity.

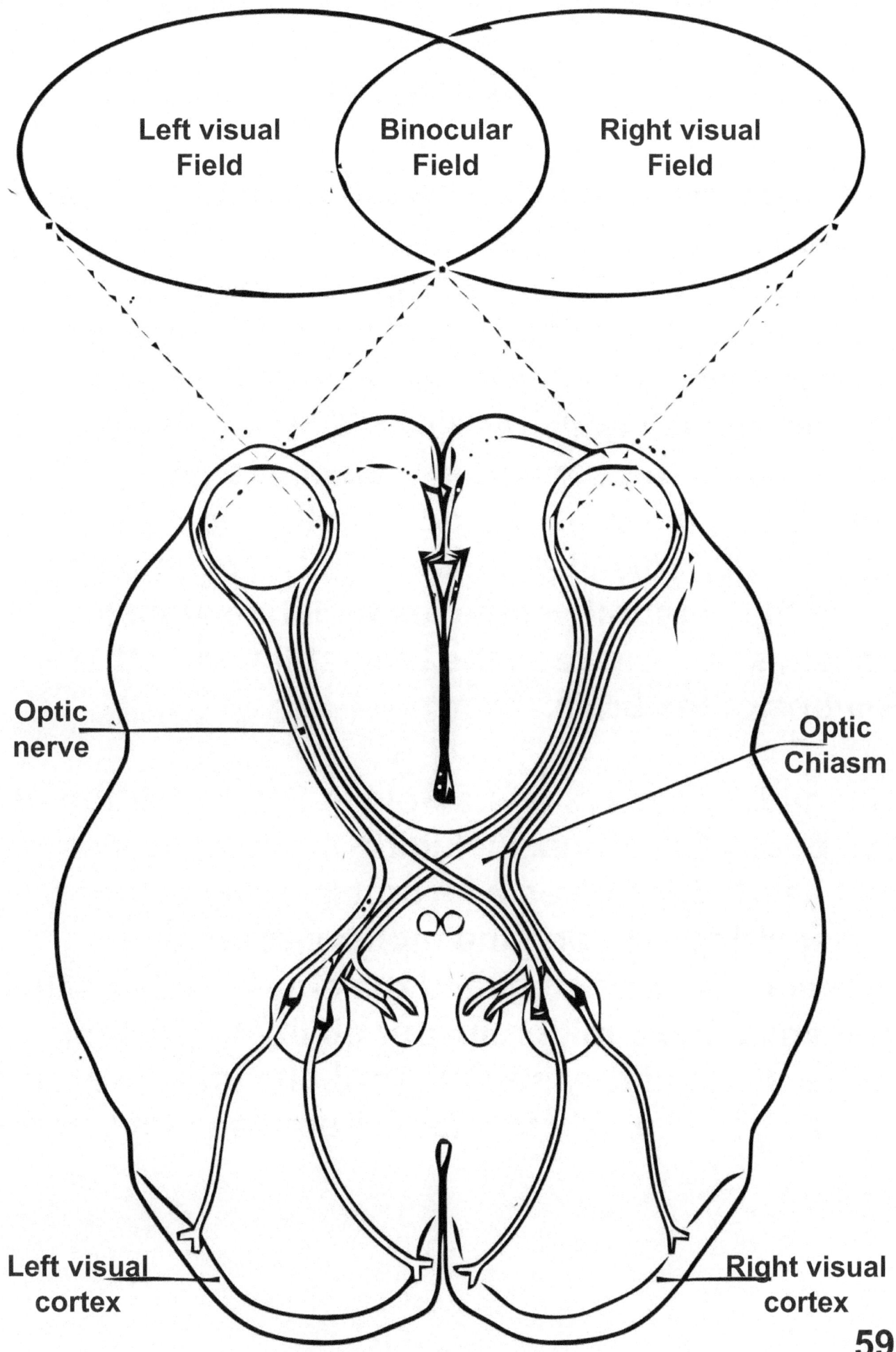

Left visual
Field

Binocular
Field

Right visual
Field

Optic
nerve

Optic
Chiasm

Left visual
cortex

Right visual
cortex

Visual Pathways

Midbrain

The midbrain, situated between the hindbrain and forebrain, is an integral component of the brain despite its small size. It comprises various structures, each with its own specific functions. Among these structures, the substantia nigra stands out as highly recognized. It serves as a dopamine producer and is indispensable in controlling movement. Additionally, the red nucleus plays a vital role in regulating limb movements, while the cerebral peduncles facilitate signal transmission between the brainstem and other regions of the brain.

The midbrain plays a vital role in the regulation of key bodily functions, including movement, vision, and hearing. It serves as a crucial relay center for transmitting sensory and motor information between the brainstem and thalamus. Without the presence of the midbrain, our ability to process visual and auditory stimuli would be impaired, as well as our capacity to execute precise movements.

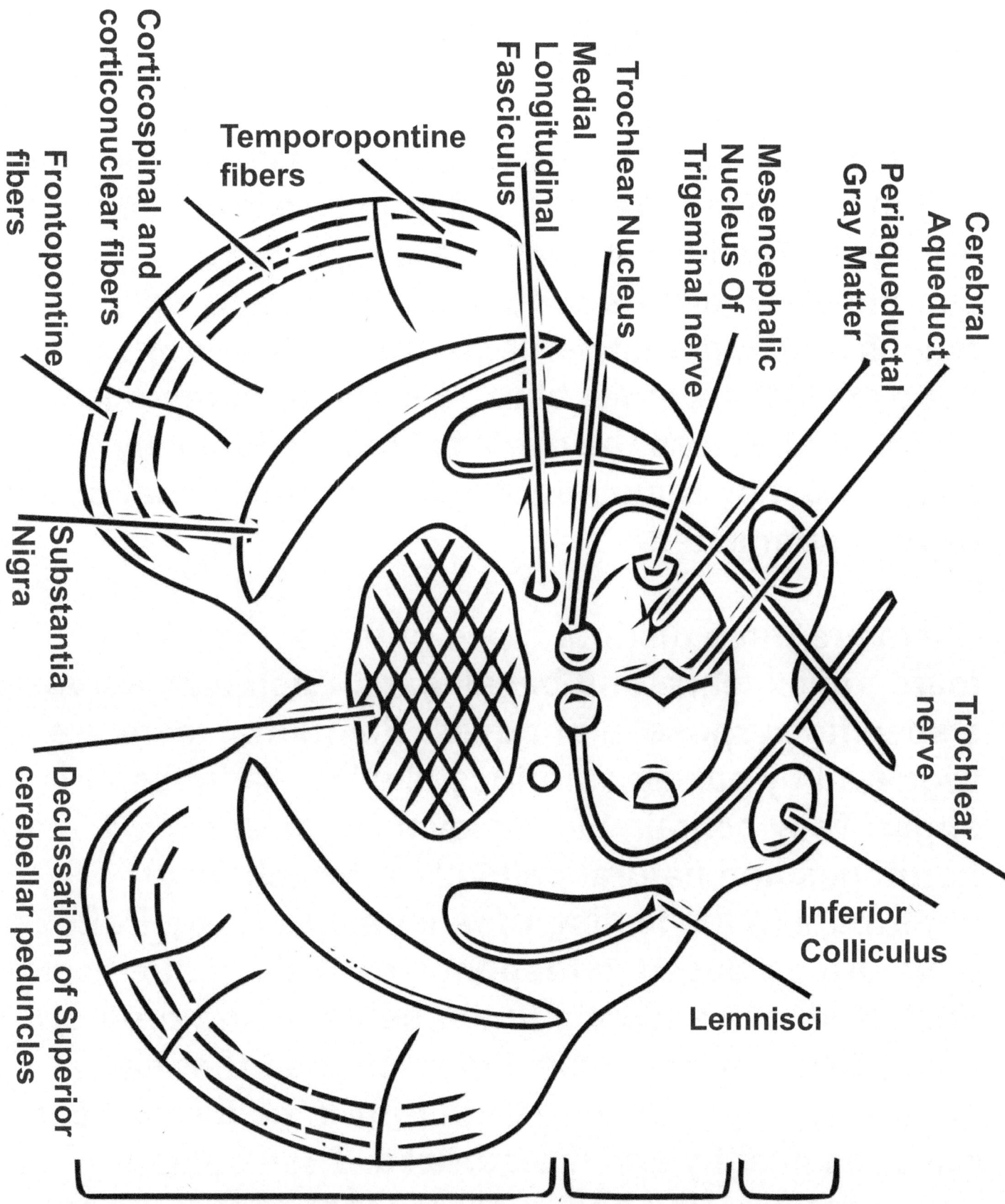

Corticospinal and
corticonuclear fibers

Temporopontine
fibers

Medial
Longitudinal
Fasciculus

Trochlear Nucleus

Mesencephalic
Nucleus Of
Trigeminal nerve

Periaqueductal
Gray Matter

Cerebral
Aqueduct

Frontopontine
fibers

Substantia
Nigra

Decussation of Superior
cerebellar peduncles

Trochlear
nerve

Inferior
Colliculus

Lemnisci

Crus Cerebri

Tegmentum

Tectum

Midbrain
cross section

61

Lacrimal Gland

The lacrimal glands, also known as tear glands, play a vital role in maintaining the moisture and health of our eyes. Positioned above each eye, these almond-sized glands produce a mixture of water, mucus, and oils that serve to protect and lubricate the eye. Whenever we blink, this blend of tears is distributed across the eye's surface, effectively cleansing it by removing any dirt or debris that could have accumulated.

There are three distinct types of tears: emotional tears, reflex tears, and basal tears. Each type serves a specific purpose in our eyes. Emotional tears are triggered by strong emotions like joy, sadness, or anger. They contain higher levels of stress hormones and natural painkillers, which may contribute to the feeling of relief after crying. Reflex tears are produced in response to irritants such as dust or smoke and help flush them out and protect the eye from harm. Basal tears, on the other hand, are constantly produced throughout the day to keep our eyes healthy and moisturized. They contain important proteins and nutrients that contribute to eye health and lubrication.

Tear film

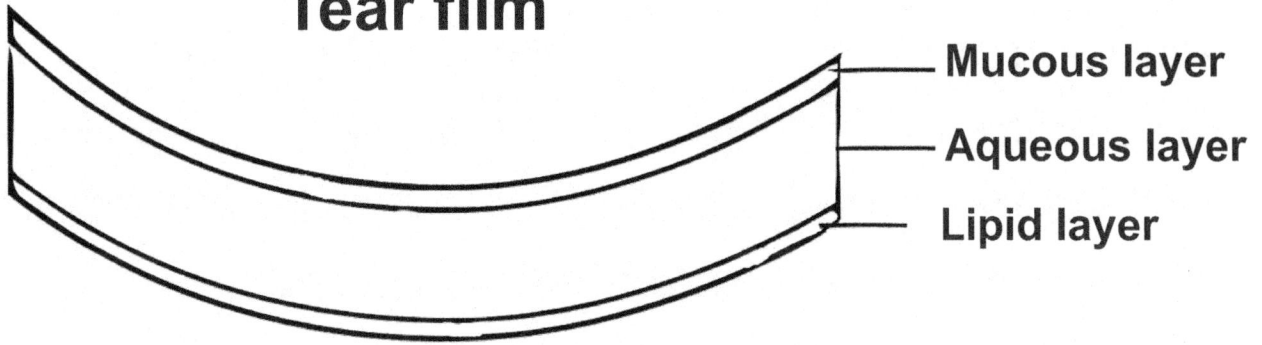

- Mucous layer
- Aqueous layer
- Lipid layer

Tear gland

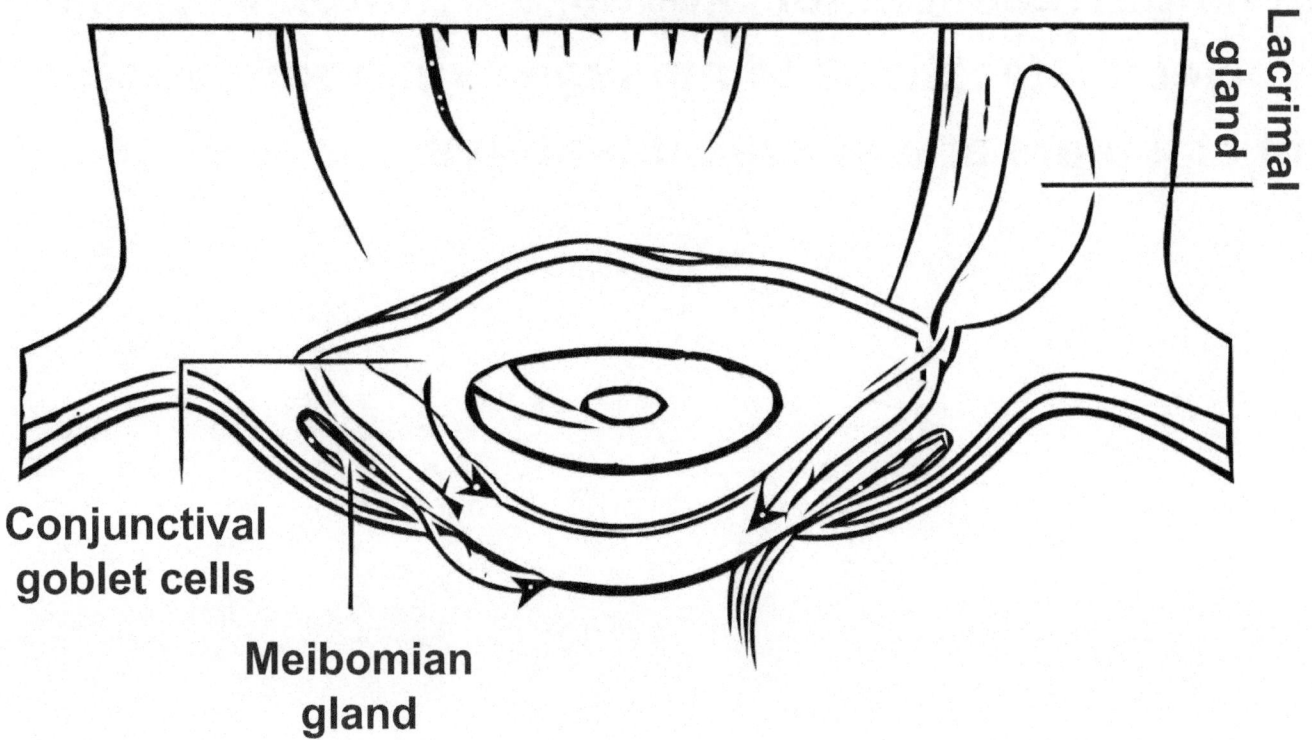

Lacrimal gland

Conjunctival goblet cells

Meibomian gland

<u>**Dry eye syndrome**</u> is a common disorder that occurs when tears aren't able to provide adequate lubrication for the eyes. Symptoms of dry eye syndrome include stinging or burning in the eyes, blurred vision, and sensitivity to light. Treatments for dry eye syndrome include artificial tears, prescription eye drops, and in severe cases, surgery.

Sjogren's syndrome is an autoimmune disorder that affects the body's ability to produce moisture, including tears. Symptoms of Sjogren's syndrome include dry mouth and eyes, fatigue, joint pain, and swelling. Treatment for Sjogren's syndrome typically involves medications to manage symptoms, such as artificial tears and saliva substitutes.

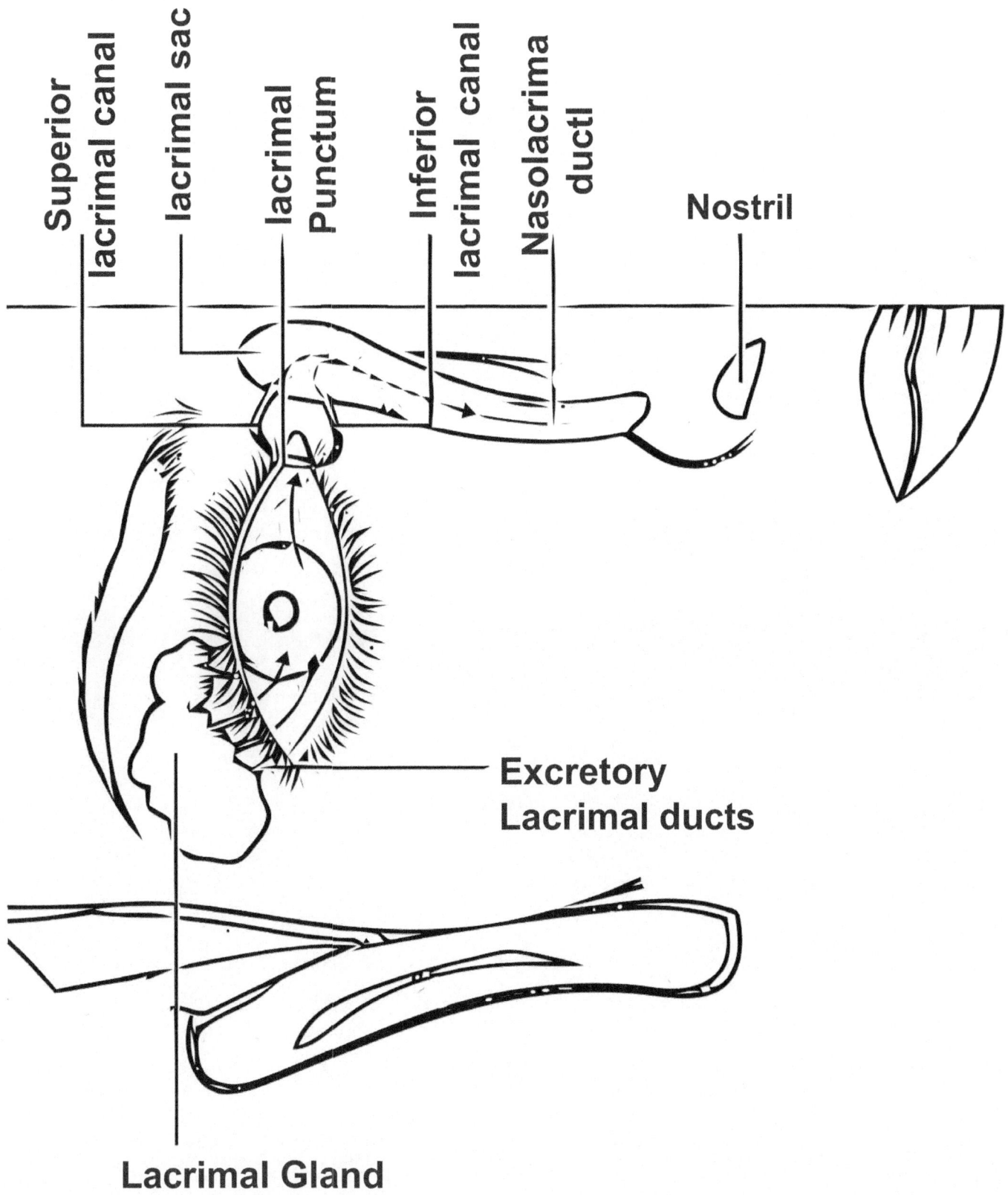

Superior
lacrimal canal

lacrimal sac

lacrimal
Punctum

Inferior
lacrimal canal

Nasolacrima
ductl

Nostril

Excretory
Lacrimal ducts

Lacrimal Gland

LACRIMAL
SAC

LACRIMAL
GLAND

BLOCKAGE

NASOLACRIMAL
DUCT

EXCESSIVE TEARING
AND EYE MUCUS
DISCHARGE

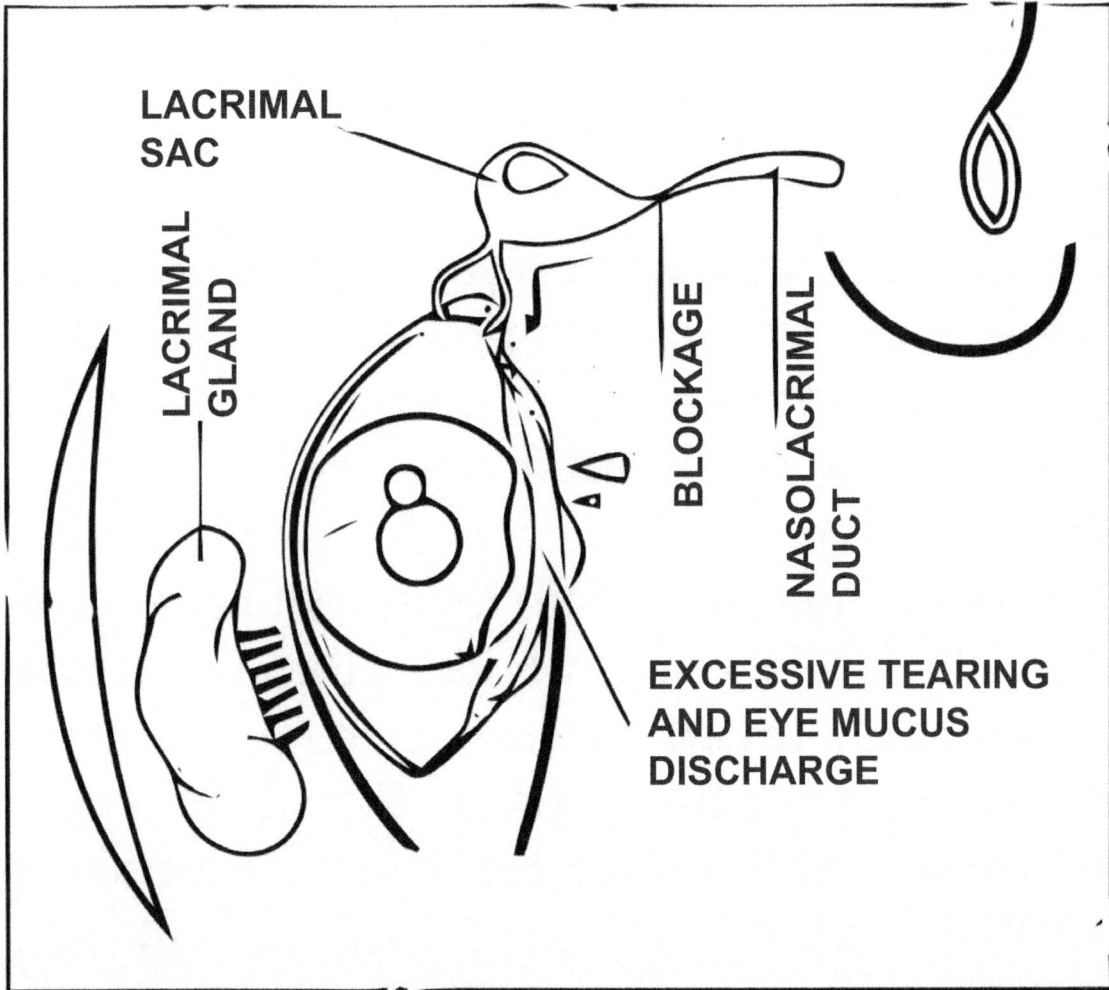

BLOCKED TEAR DUCT

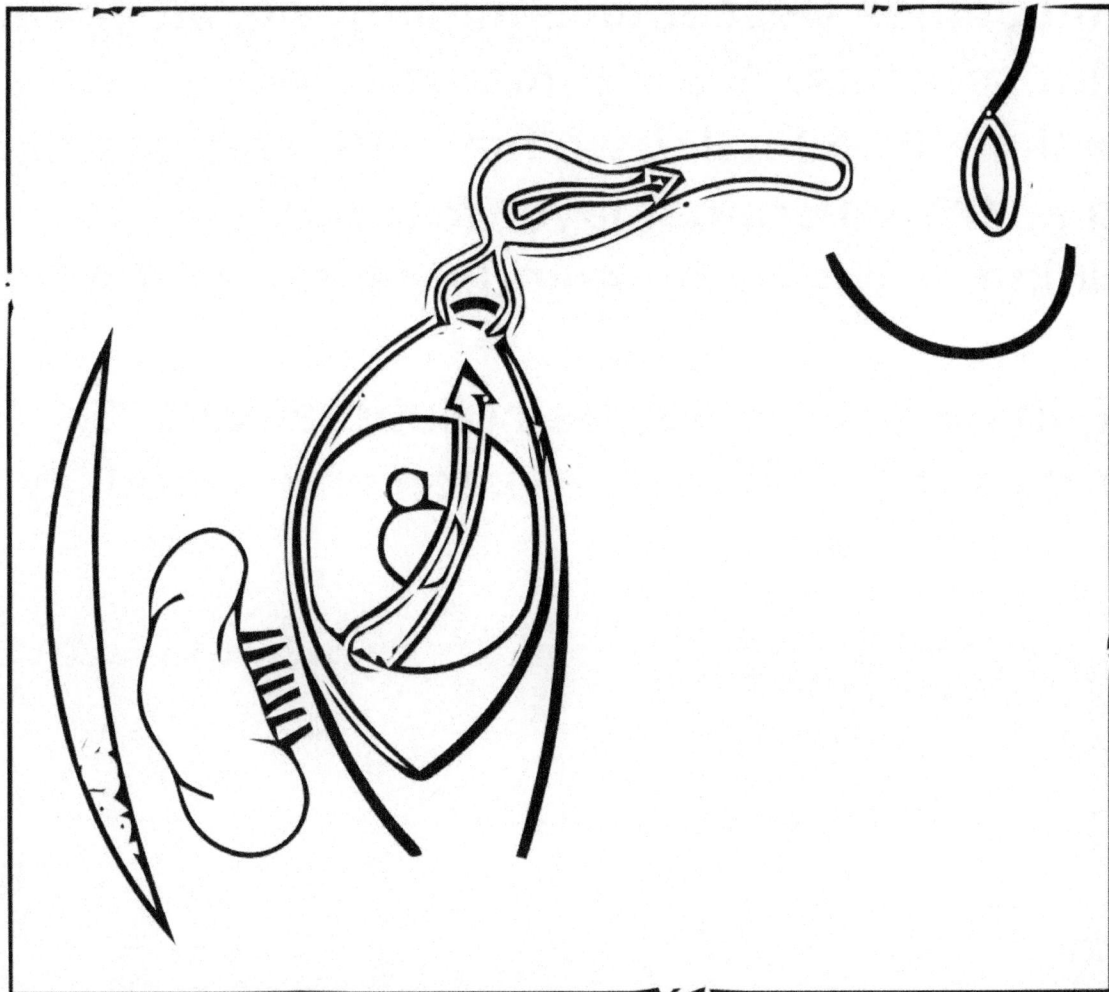

NORMAL TEAR DRAINAGE

Cornea

The cornea, the transparent outer layer of the eye, is responsible for covering and protecting the iris, pupil, and anterior chamber. It consists of five layers that work together to maintain the health and function of the eye.

Firstly, there is the epithelium layer, which acts as a shield against foreign objects like dust and bacteria. Next is Bowman's layer, a thin but crucial fibrous support structure for the cornea. The stroma comes next and serves as the thickest layer composed of strong collagen fibers that contribute to both its strength and transparency.

After that comes Descemet's membrane, an elastic layer that separates the stroma from the endothelium. And finally, we have the endothelium, serving as the innermost layer responsible for maintaining clarity by pumping fluid out of the stroma.

Overall, these distinct layers collaboratively contribute to ensuring clear vision and overall eye health.

Cornea structure

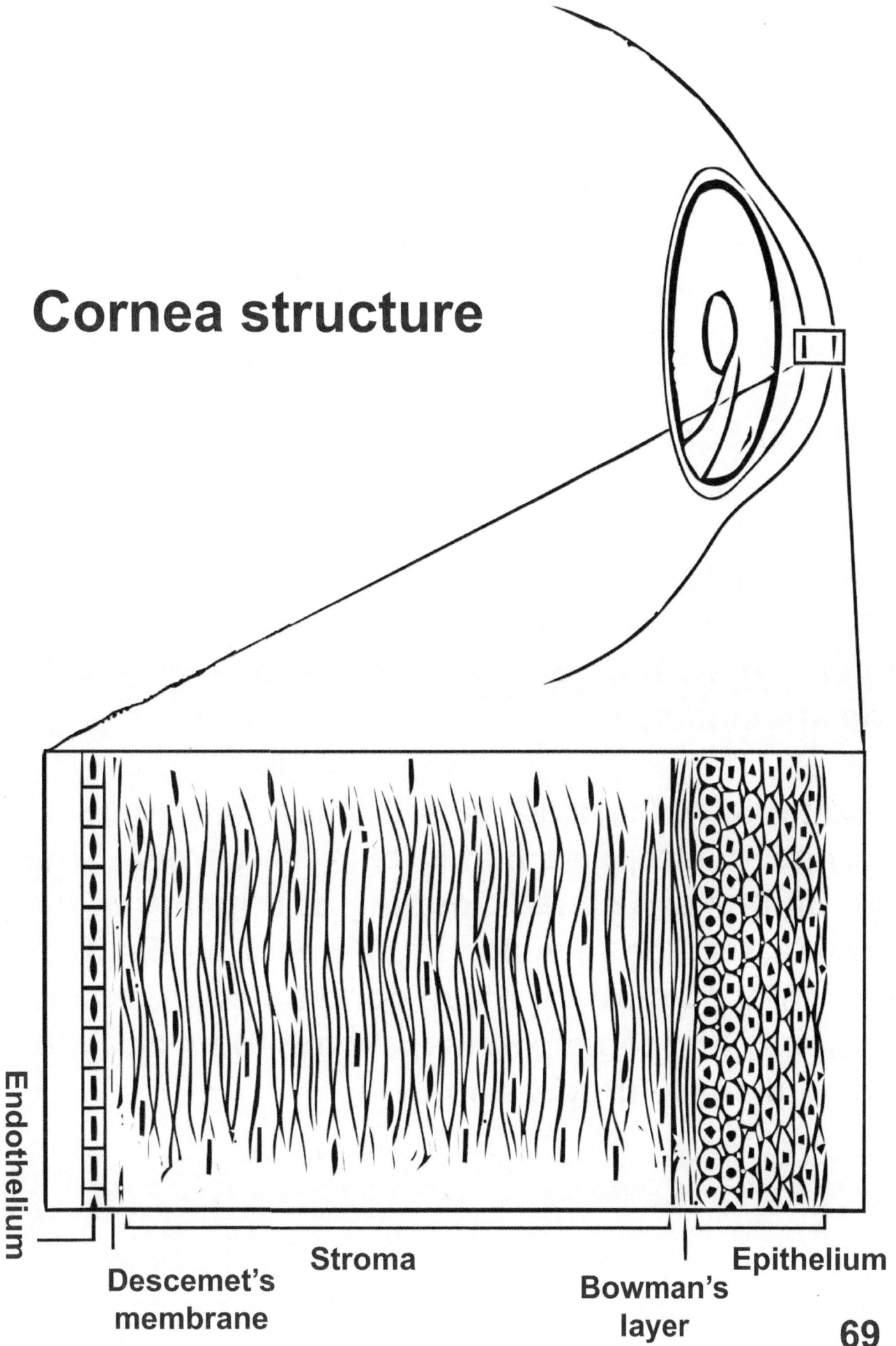

Endothelium

Descemet's membrane

Stroma

Bowman's layer

Epithelium

69

Corneal abrasions are a prevalent issue that affects the cornea. They occur when the surface of the cornea is scratched, often by objects like fingernails or foreign bodies. While they may seem insignificant, corneal abrasions can cause intense pain and potentially lead to serious complications if left untreated.

Another common problem is corneal infections, which can cause substantial damage to the eye. These infections are typically caused by bacteria, viruses, or fungi and can result in vision loss if not promptly addressed. Symptoms of a corneal infection include redness, pain, and discharge from the affected eye.

Additionally, there are genetic disorders known as corneal dystrophies that impact the cornea. These conditions can cause clouding or thinning of the cornea, leading to vision impairment. While there is currently no cure for these conditions, treatment options exist to help manage symptoms and slow down disease progression.

Abrasion

Cornea

Abrasion

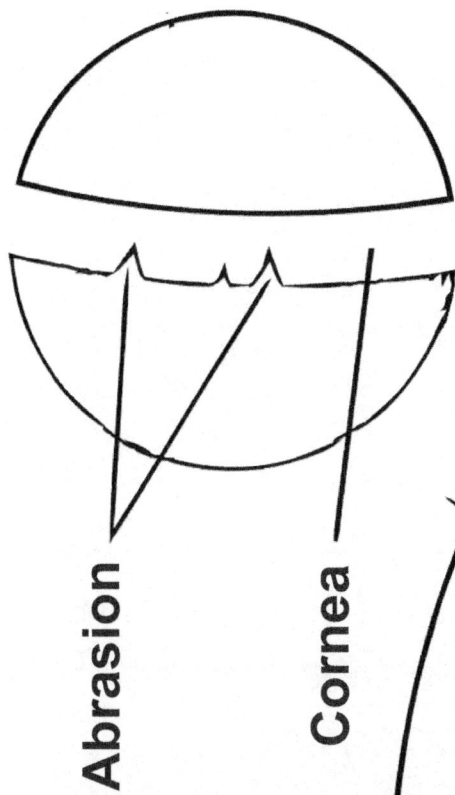

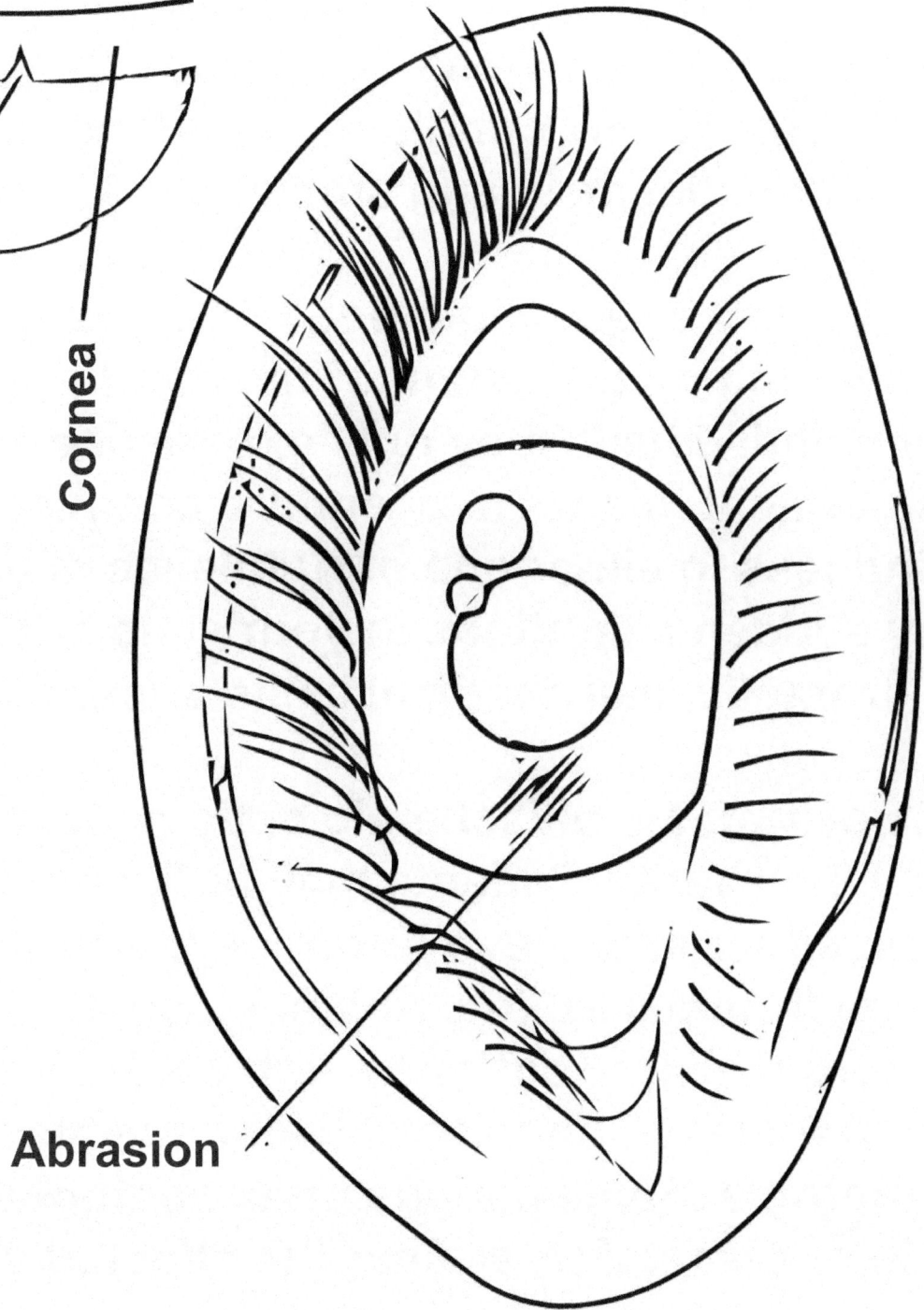

Cornea abrasion

71

Ischemic optic neuropathy

Ischemic optic neuropathy is a medical condition characterized by insufficient blood flow to the optic nerve, leading to potential nerve damage and subsequent vision loss. Numerous factors can contribute to this condition, including high blood pressure, diabetes, and smoking.

The impact of ischemic optic neuropathy varies depending on the extent of the condition. While some individuals may only experience minor vision impairment, others may endure complete blindness in either one or both eyes. If you notice any sudden alterations in your vision, it is crucial to promptly seek medical assistance.

The symptoms of ischemic optic neuropathy can vary in severity. Patients may notice sudden vision loss, either in one eye or both eyes, which can range from partial to complete loss. Blurred or distorted vision, difficulty with color perception, and decreased peripheral vision are also possible symptoms. Some patients may additionally feel pain or discomfort around the affected eye, particularly when moving it.

In more severe cases, patients may even experience visual hallucinations or temporary episodes of blindness. It is crucial to understand that not all individuals with ischemic optic neuropathy will have the same symptoms, and some might not experience any at all. If you notice any changes in your vision, it is imperative to seek immediate medical attention.

The diagnosis of ischemic optic neuropathy involves a thorough assessment of the patient's medical history, physical examination, and various diagnostic tests. To gather important information, the doctor will inquire about the patient's symptoms, medical background, and current medications. Additionally, a comprehensive eye exam will be conducted to evaluate visual acuity, visual fields, and examine the optic nerve.

To confirm a diagnosis of ischemic optic neuropathy, several diagnostic tests may be utilized. These include optical coherence tomography (OCT), fluorescein angiography, and magnetic resonance imaging (MRI). OCT employs light waves to generate detailed images of the retina and optic nerve. Fluorescein angiography involves injecting a specialized dye into the patient's bloodstream and capturing photographs as it circulates through the blood vessels in the eye. MRI provides highly detailed images of both the brain and optic nerve.

The appropriate treatment for ischemic optic neuropathy depends on factors such as underlying causes and disease severity. In some instances, spontaneous resolution may occur without intervention. However, if significant vision loss or severe symptoms are present, treatment may be required. Treatment options may involve medications aimed at improving blood flow to the optic nerve like corticosteroids or anticoagulants or surgical procedures to alleviate pressure on the optic nerve.

While there is currently no cure for ischemic optic neuropathy, early detection and prompt treatment can aid in preventing further deterioration of vision.

Ischemic Optic Neuropathy

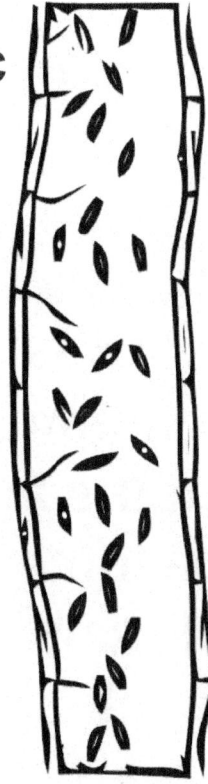

Impaired blood flow

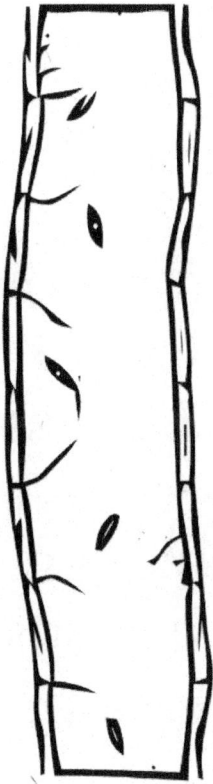

Normal blood flow

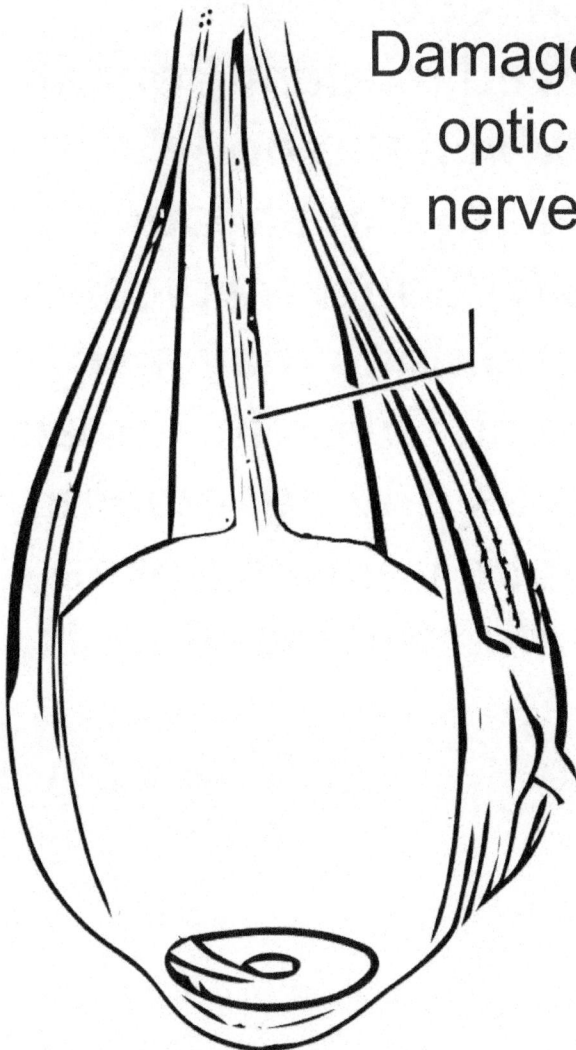

Damaged optic nerve

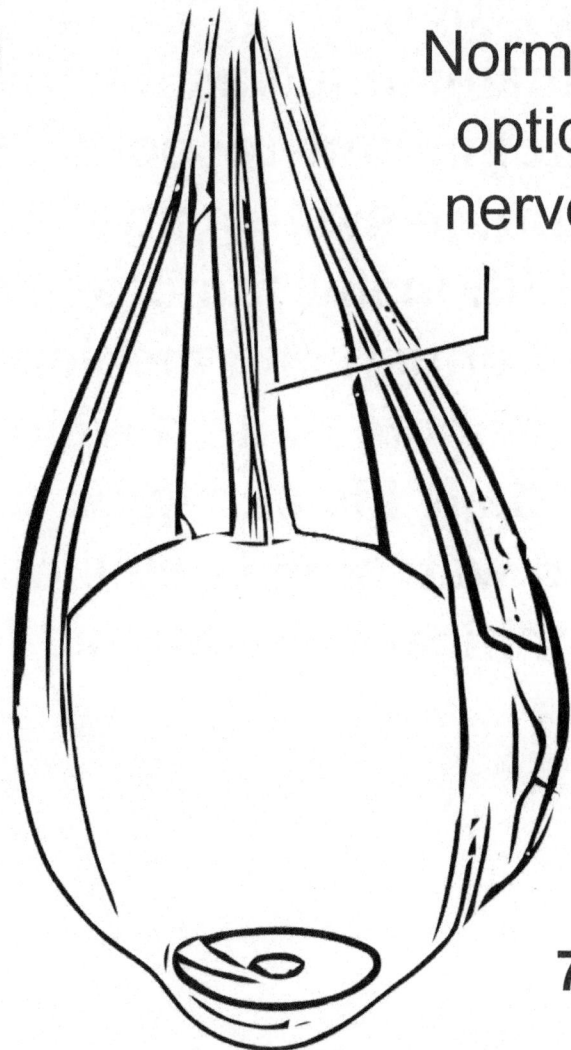

Normal optic nerve

75

Optic Neuritis

Optic neuritis is a condition that affects the optic nerve, an essential component for transmitting visual information from the eye to the brain. This occurs when the myelin, a protective covering of the nerve, becomes inflamed or damaged. As a result, individuals may experience a range of symptoms such as blurred vision, loss of color vision, and eye pain.

Although the exact cause of optic neuritis remains unclear, it is believed to stem from an autoimmune response in which the body's immune system attacks the myelin sheath. Additionally, factors like infections, medications, and underlying medical conditions may also contribute to its development. Given its impact on daily life activities such as driving, reading, and watching television, optic neuritis poses significant challenges for affected individuals.

Optic neuritis is a medical condition that affects the optic nerve, which is responsible for transmitting visual information from the eye to the brain. The most prevalent symptom of optic neuritis is blurred vision, which can significantly impair activities such as reading, driving, and performing daily tasks. Additional symptoms may include a loss of color vision, eye pain, and sensitivity to light. These symptoms can have a significant impact on an individual's everyday life, hindering their ability to work, socialize, and engage in hobbies.

The severity and duration of these symptoms can vary among individuals. While some may only experience mild symptoms that subside naturally over time, others may experience more severe symptoms that necessitate medical intervention. It is crucial to seek immediate medical attention if you encounter any of these symptoms since early diagnosis and treatment are vital in preventing permanent vision loss.

The diagnosis of optic neuritis usually involves a series of visual tests and imaging techniques. Visual tests may consist of assessing visual acuity, color vision, and conducting visual field testing. In addition, MRI scans can be employed to identify any inflammation in the optic nerve.

Timely identification of optic neuritis is vital for effective treatment and care. If you encounter signs such as blurred vision, diminished color perception, or eye discomfort, it is crucial to promptly seek medical assistance.

Optic neuritis is a medical condition that affects the optic nerve, which is responsible for transmitting visual information from the eye to the brain. Although there is currently no known cure for optic neuritis, there are several treatment options available that can effectively manage its symptoms and prevent further damage to the optic nerve.

One commonly used treatment method for optic neuritis is steroid therapy. This involves administering high doses of corticosteroids to reduce inflammation in the optic nerve. Through this approach, vision can be significantly improved, and the risk of future episodes of optic neuritis can be minimized.

In addition to steroid therapy, immunosuppressive drugs like azathioprine and mycophenolate may also be prescribed. These medications work by suppressing the immune system and reducing inflammation in the optic nerve. Their use has been found to be beneficial in managing optic neuritis symptoms.

Depending on individual circumstances, other medications such as pain relievers or anti-seizure drugs may also be prescribed to address specific symptoms associated with optic neuritis.

It's important to note that any treatment plan should be customized based on an individual's specific needs and under medical supervision. Therefore, consulting with a healthcare professional is crucial for determining the most appropriate course of action when it comes to managing optic neuritis.

Normal

Optic Neuritis

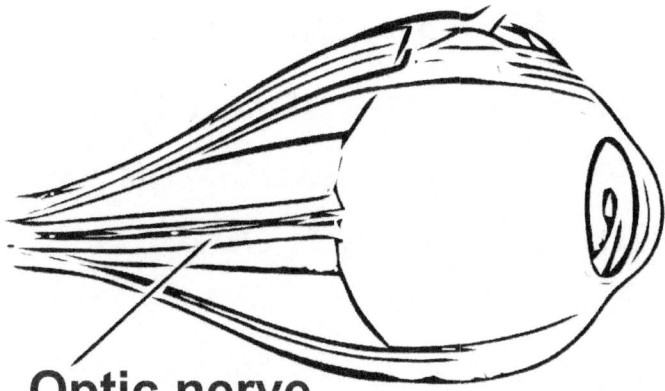

Optic nerve

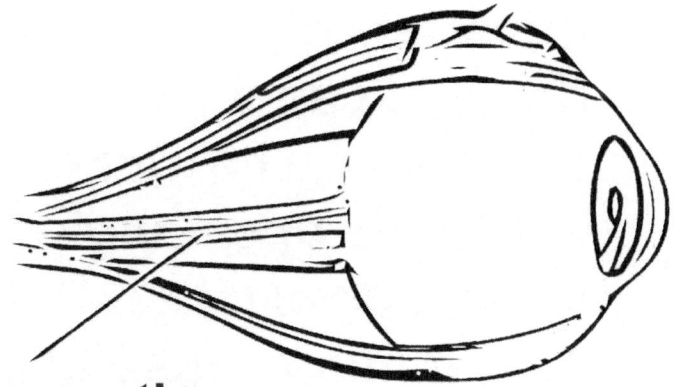

Inflammation of optic nerve

Myelin sheath

Damaged myelin

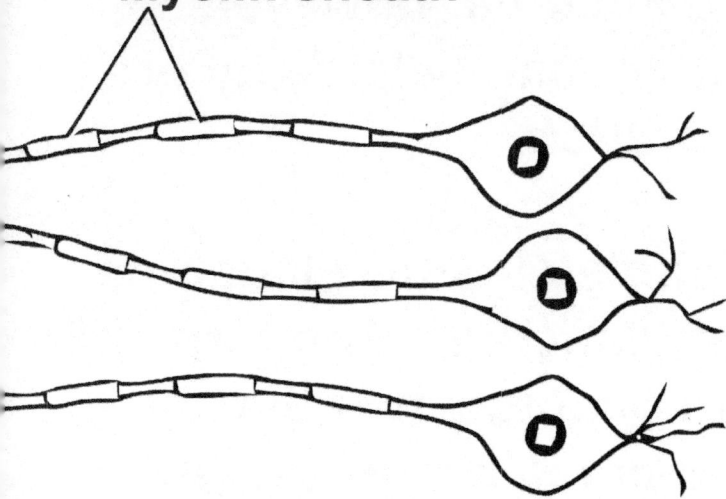

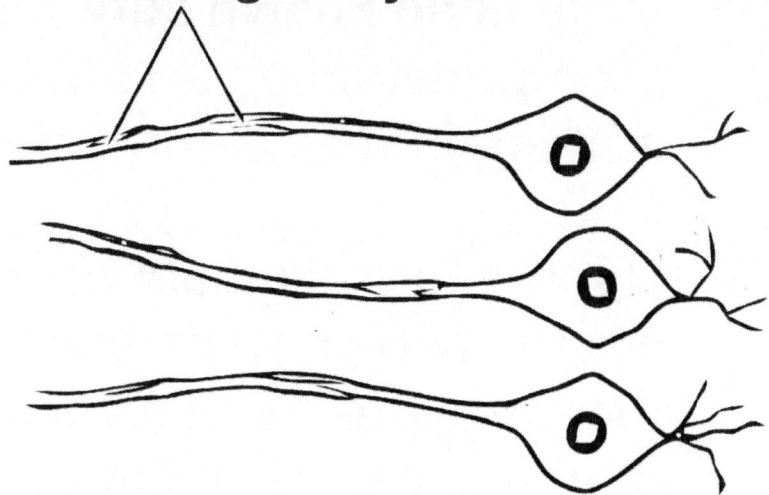

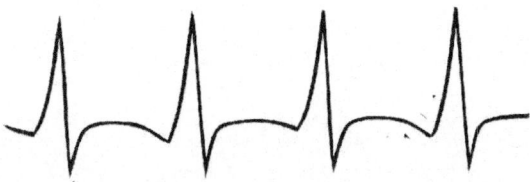

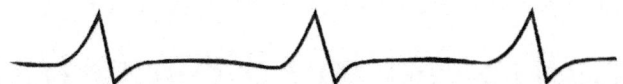

Glaucoma

Is a collection of eye disorders that harm the optic nerve, responsible for transmitting visual information to the brain. Without treatment, this damage can result in vision impairment or complete blindness. The most prevalent form of glaucoma is known as open-angle glaucoma, although other variations exist.

The primary cause of glaucoma is heightened pressure within the eye, often due to fluid buildup. However, certain individuals may develop glaucoma even without elevated eye pressure. Regrettably, there is no known cure for glaucoma; however, prompt detection and treatment can help delay or halt additional vision deterioration.

Open-angle glaucoma and angle-closure glaucoma are the two primary types of glaucoma. The former is the more prevalent form and occurs when the drainage canals in the eye become progressively blocked, leading to increased pressure. Conversely, angle-closure glaucoma arises when the iris is positioned too closely to the drainage canals, hindering fluid flow and causing sudden pressure spikes.

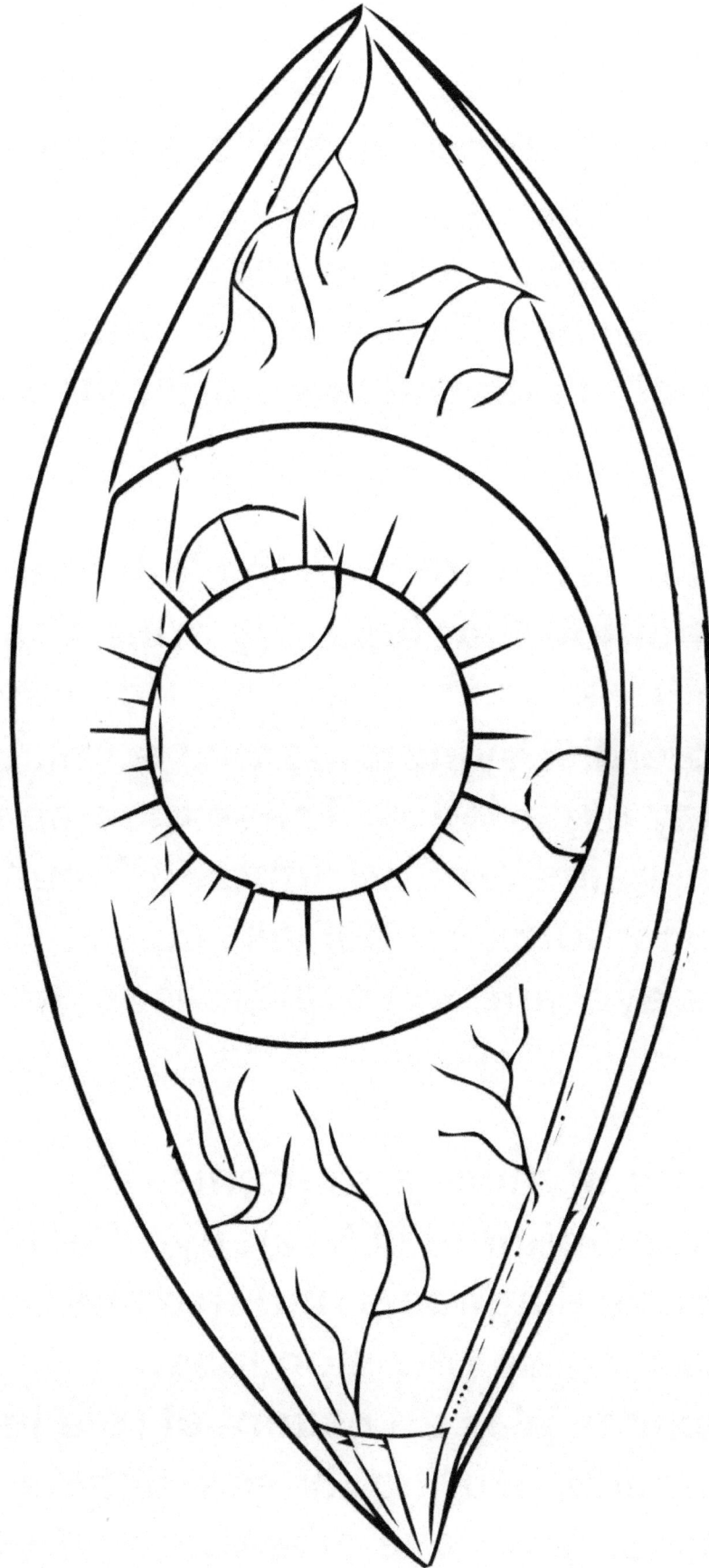

GLAUCOMA

There are also secondary variants of glaucoma that can arise from other medical conditions or medication usage. These include pigmentary glaucoma, uveitic glaucoma, and steroid-induced glaucoma. Each type of glaucoma possesses distinct characteristics and necessitates tailored treatment approaches. Close collaboration with your doctor is crucial to determine an optimal course of action.

Glaucoma, often referred to as the 'silent thief of sight,' is a condition that typically doesn't show any symptoms until vision loss occurs. However, there are several potential symptoms that some individuals may experience. These include blurred or hazy vision, halos around lights, difficulty seeing in low light conditions, tunnel vision, eye pain, redness in the eye, and in severe cases, nausea and vomiting.

If you notice any of these symptoms, it's crucial to schedule an appointment with an eye doctor as soon as possible. Early diagnosis and treatment can greatly reduce the risk of vision loss.
Regular eye exams play an essential role in detecting glaucoma. During these exams, your eye doctor will assess your eye pressure and examine

GLAUCOMA

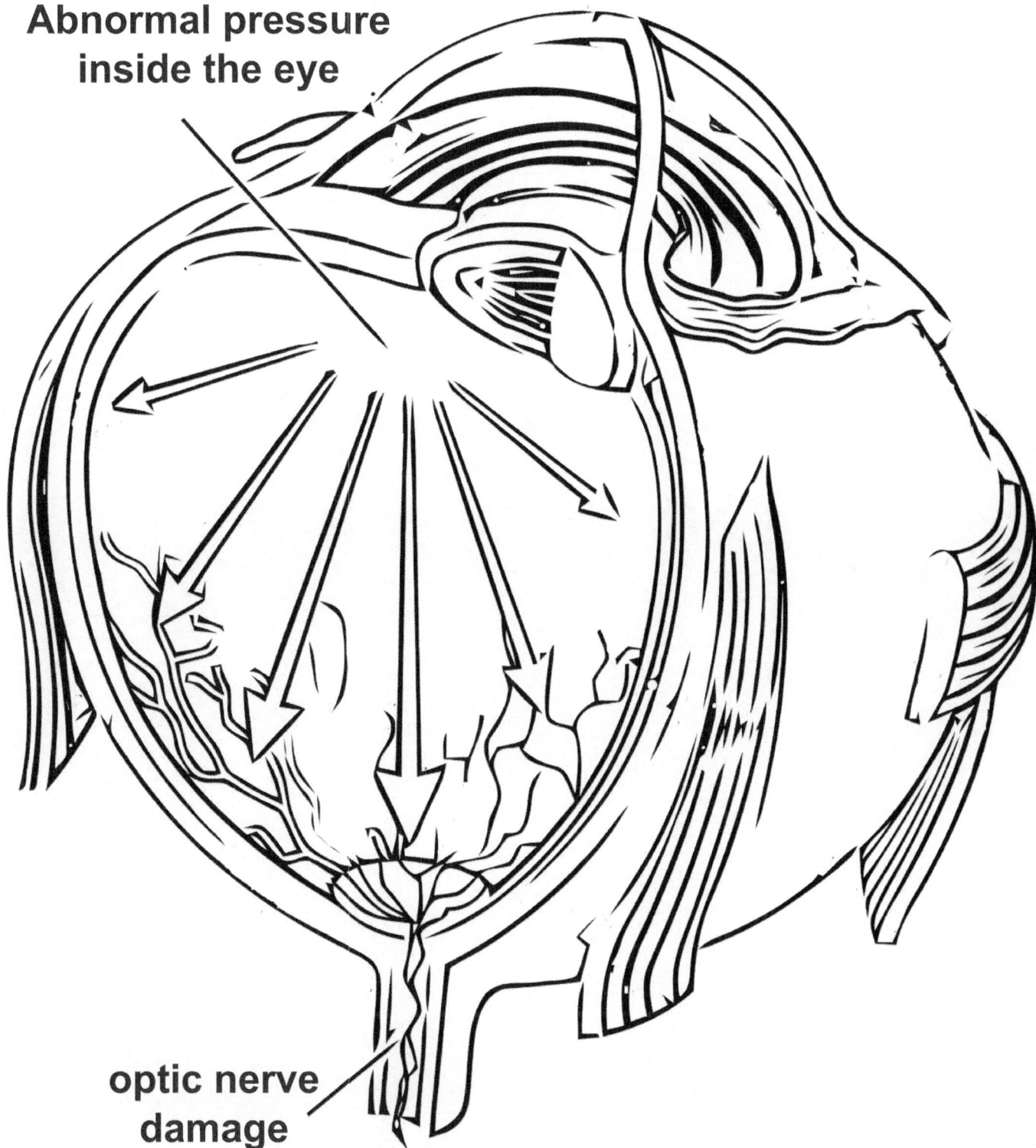

Abnormal pressure
inside the eye

optic nerve
damage

your optic nerve for any signs of damage. By staying vigilant with routine check-ups, you can take proactive steps towards maintaining healthy eyesight.

There are various risk factors that are associated with glaucoma, including age, family history, ethnicity, and certain medical conditions. As we get older, our likelihood of developing glaucoma increases. Furthermore, if a member of our family has had glaucoma, it raises the probability of us developing the condition as well. Certain ethnic groups such as African Americans and Hispanics also have a higher risk for glaucoma. Lastly, medical conditions like diabetes and high blood pressure can elevate our risk for glaucoma.

Although these risk factors cannot be completely eliminated, there are measures we can take to manage them effectively. Regular eye examinations play a vital role in early detection of glaucoma, especially if any of the aforementioned risk factors apply to us. In addition to that, adopting a healthy lifestyle by incorporating regular exercise, maintaining a balanced diet, and effectively managing any underlying medical conditions can significantly reduce our risk for glaucoma.

Treatment

There are a variety of treatment options available for glaucoma, ranging from eye drops to laser therapy and surgery. Eye drops are often prescribed as the initial treatment, as they effectively lower intraocular pressure (IOP) by regulating fluid production or improving fluid drainage within the eye. It is important to note that eye drops may have some side effects, including stinging sensation, redness, and temporary blurred vision.

Laser therapy is another viable option that can be employed to reduce IOP by enhancing the drainage system in the eye. This procedure is typically swift and painless; however, multiple sessions may be required over time to maintain its effectiveness. For certain patients with advanced stages of glaucoma, surgery might be recommended. There are various surgical interventions available, each accompanied by its own set of advantages and potential risks.

Glaucoma

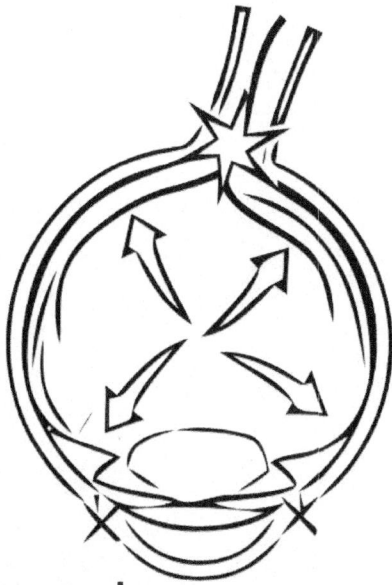

**Increased
pressure**

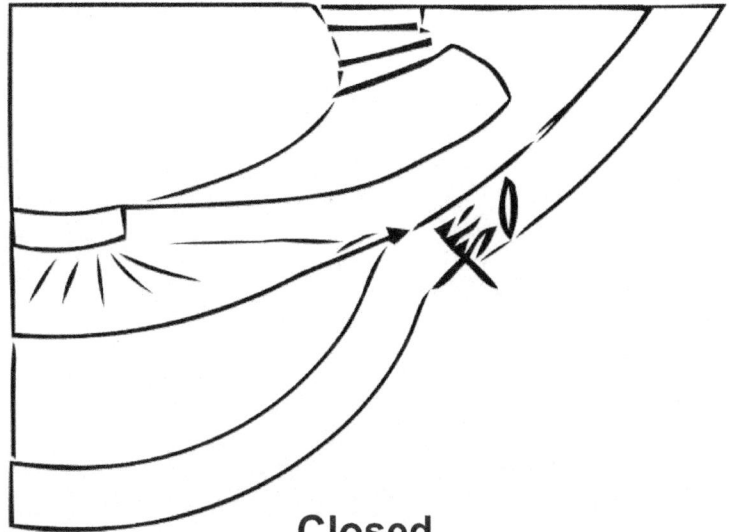

**Closed
angle**

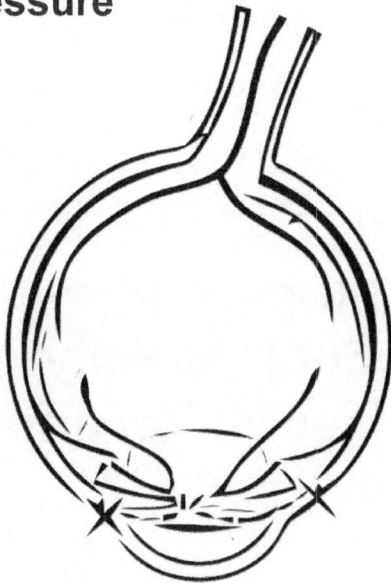

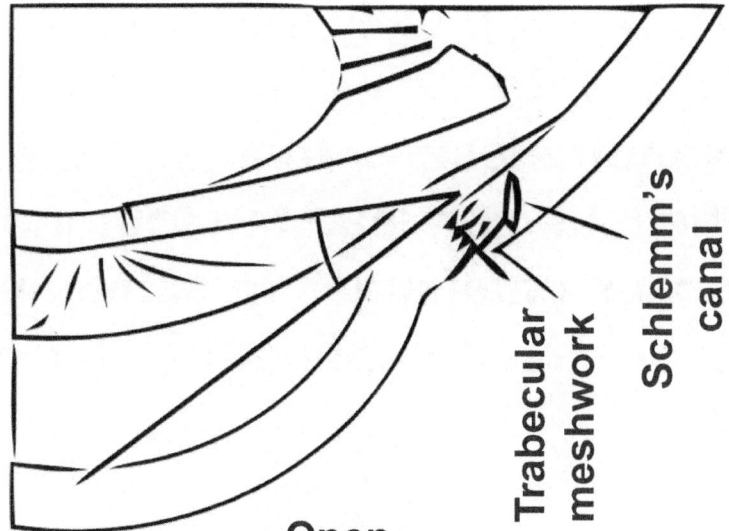

**Open
angle**

Trabecular
meshwork

Schlemm's
canal

Healthy Eye

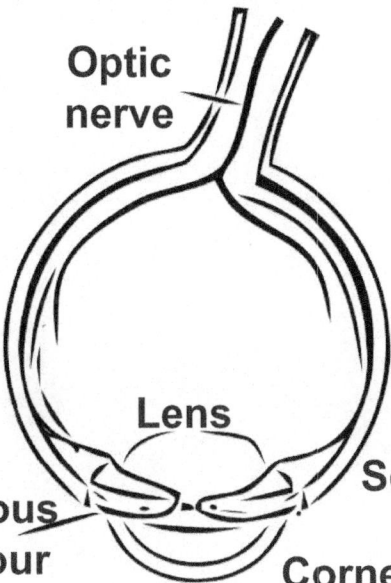

**Optic
nerve**

Lens

**Aqueous
Humour**

**Schlemm's
canal**

Cornea

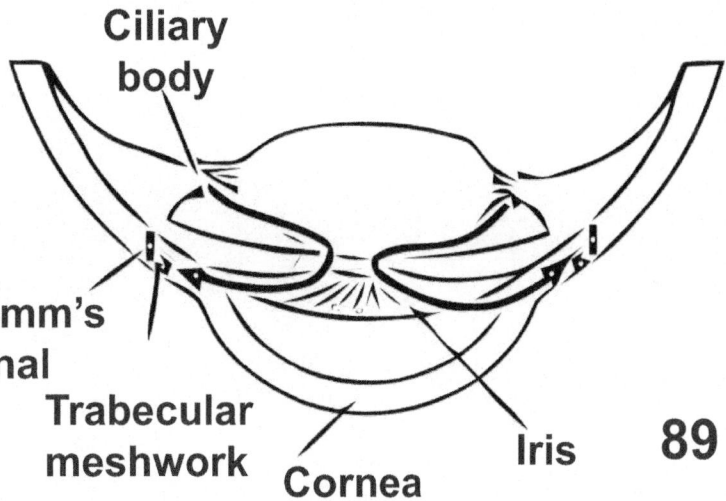

**Ciliary
body**

**Trabecular
meshwork**

Cornea

Iris

89

Cataract

Cataract, a prevalent eye condition that impacts countless individuals globally, arises when the eye's lens becomes opaque, resulting in impaired vision. Typically clear, the lens aids in directing light onto the retina situated at the back of the eye. Nonetheless, with age, protein aggregation within the lens can lead to cloudiness. Such opacity poses challenges in achieving clear vision and may even result in blindness if unaddressed.

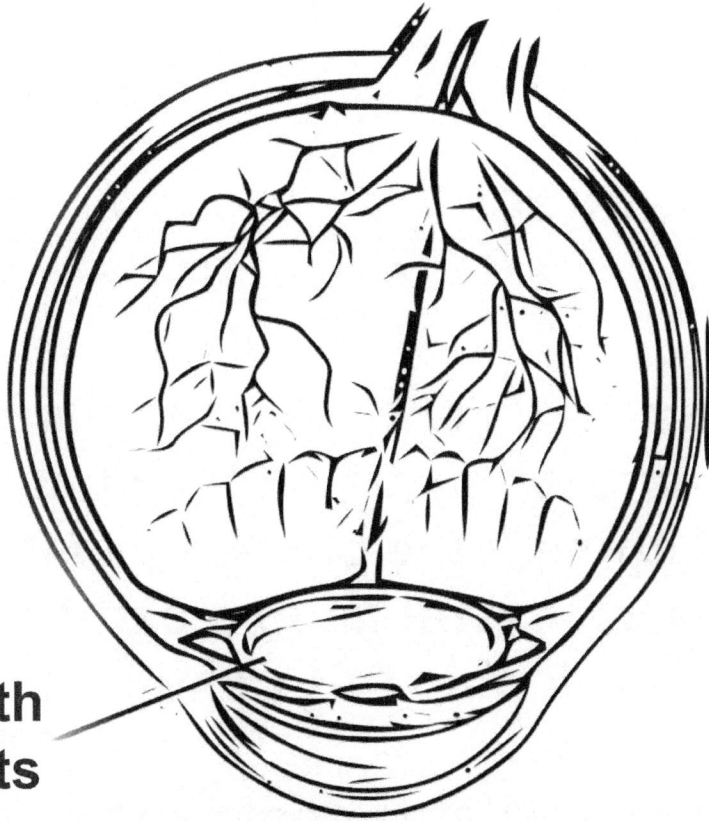

Lens with Cataracts

Cataracts

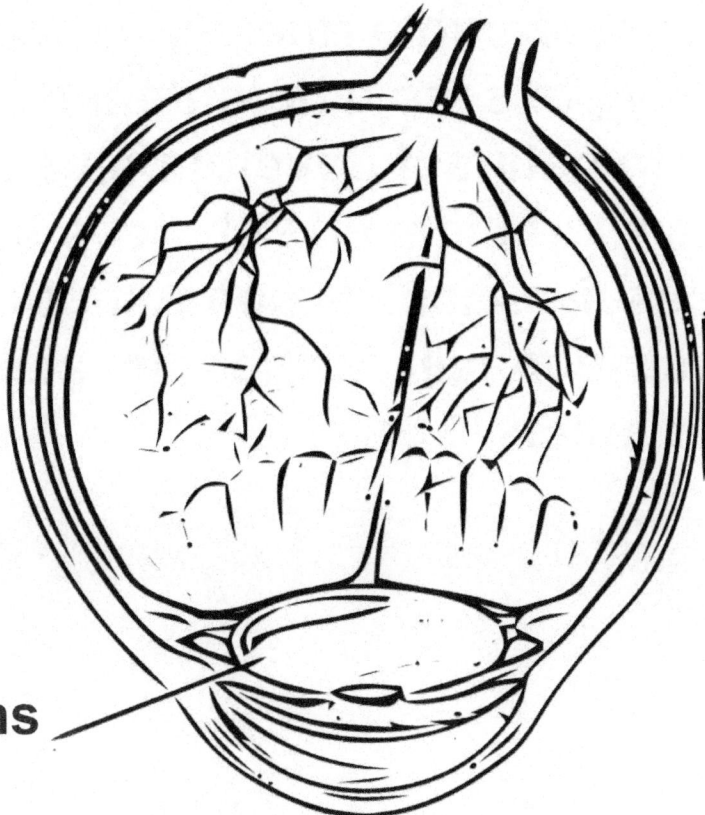

Healthy lens

Causes of Cataract

Cataracts are a prevalent eye condition with global implications, impacting a significant number of individuals. Although the precise cause of cataracts remains unclear, several factors can heighten the likelihood of developing this condition.

Perhaps the most notable contributor to cataract formation is aging. As we progress in years, proteins within our eyes have a tendency to aggregate, manifesting as hazy regions on the lens and hindering visual acuity. Genetic predisposition also plays a considerable role, as certain individuals may possess a heightened susceptibility to cataract development compared to others. Furthermore, lifestyle choices such as smoking, excessive alcohol consumption, and inadequate nutrition can further elevate the risk of developing cataracts.

Blurred vision is one of the most prevalent symptoms associated with cataracts. This visual impairment can severely hinder everyday tasks such as reading, driving, and even recognizing familiar faces. Think of it as looking through a hazy window.

Another telltale sign is heightened sensitivity to light, especially intense sources like headlights or sunlight. This heightened sensitivity may lead to feelings of discomfort or even acute pain in the eyes.

Furthermore, individuals suffering from cataracts often encounter difficulties seeing clearly in low-light conditions, impacting their ability to navigate during evening hours or in dimly lit environments.

To truly grasp the impact of these symptoms on daily life, personal anecdotes and stories are invaluable tools. For instance, imagine someone sharing their heartbreaking experience of relinquishing nighttime driving privileges due to their cataracts, or detailing the struggles they faced trying to read their beloved books.

Treatment

When it comes to treating cataracts, there are two main options available: surgery and lifestyle changes. The most commonly recommended treatment is surgery, which involves the removal of the cloudy lens in the eye and replacing it with an artificial lens. This procedure has a high success rate of over 95% and is considered safe and effective. However, it's important to note that like any surgical procedure, there are potential risks involved such as infection, bleeding, and even vision loss. Before undergoing the surgery, your doctor will thoroughly discuss these risks with you.

In addition to surgery, making certain lifestyle changes can also help manage cataract symptoms. For example, wearing sunglasses that offer protection against glare can significantly reduce discomfort associated with cataracts. Using brighter lights when reading or doing close work can also prove beneficial by improving visibility. Another lifestyle adjustment would be avoiding driving at night if visibility is impaired due to cataracts.

While lifestyle changes cannot cure cataracts themselves, they can certainly enhance your overall quality of life and potentially delay the need for surgery. Combining both treatment options based on your unique circumstances may lead to optimal outcomes in managing this common eye condition.

CATARACT SURGERY

Eye with cataract

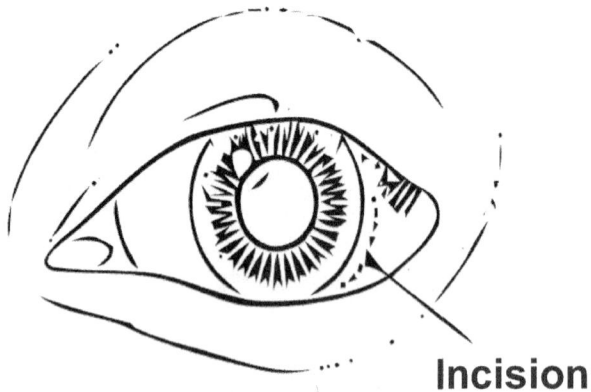

Incision

Lens implant

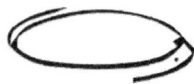

1. The diseased lens is pulled out

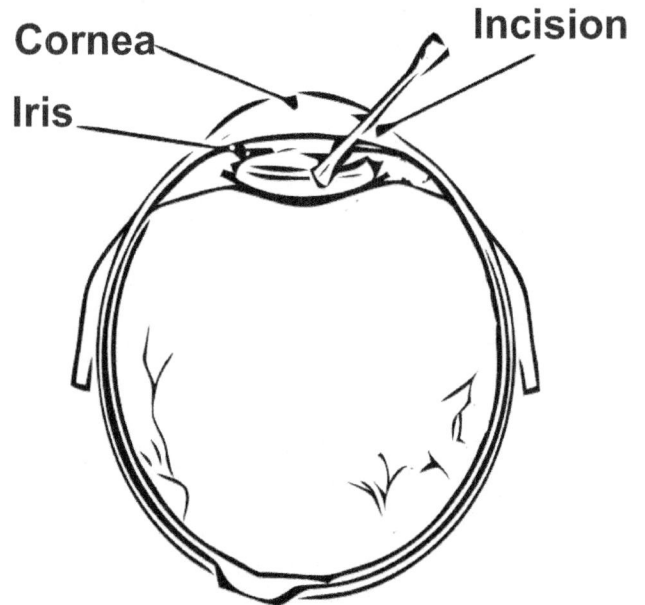

Cornea

Iris

Incision

2. Implant inserted

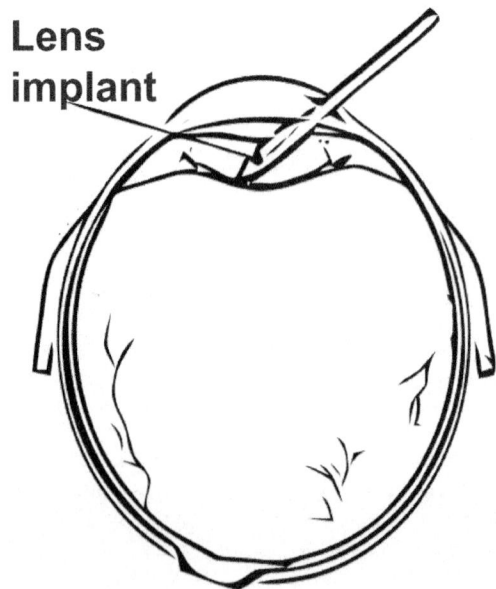

Lens implant

3. Lens implanted into position

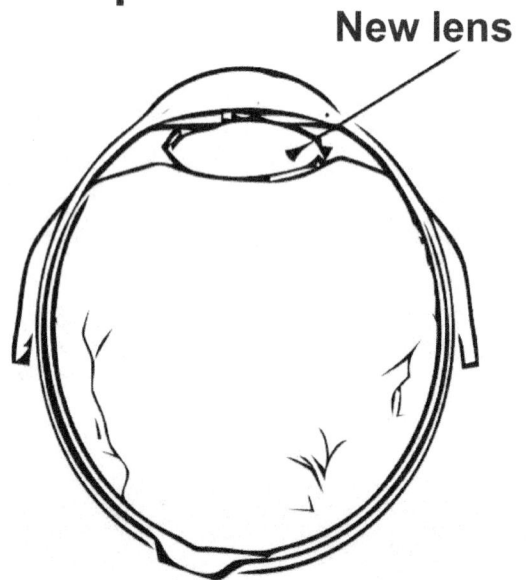

New lens

Pterygium

Pterygium is a condition characterized by the formation of abnormal tissue growth on the conjunctiva, the clear membrane that covers the white part of the eye. Although its exact cause remains unknown, pterygium development can be influenced by various factors.

Exposure to UV radiation, either from the sun or other sources, stands as one of the main contributors to pterygium. Consequently, individuals residing in sunny climates or frequently engaging in outdoor activities are more susceptible to developing this condition. Additionally, other risk factors include dry eye syndrome, exposure to dust and wind, as well as certain occupations like farming or fishing.

Pterygium, also known as surfer's eye, is a condition that involves the development of a growth on the conjunctiva, which is the thin covering over the white part of the eye. The primary indication of pterygium is redness in the affected eye, often accompanied by sensations of itching or burning. These symptoms can worsen when exposed to sunlight or wind.

As the growth progresses, it can lead to blurred vision and a sensation of having something lodged in your eye. In severe cases, pterygium can even block vision by obstructing the pupil, resulting in vision loss. If you are experiencing any of these symptoms, it is crucial to seek immediate medical attention.

There are various treatment options available for pterygium, depending on the severity of the condition. For mild cases, lubricating eye drops can provide relief from dryness and discomfort. In more severe situations, surgery may be required to eliminate the growth.

One surgical approach is known as excision with conjunctival autografting, where the pterygium is surgically removed and a healthy piece of tissue from the patient's own conjunctiva is transplanted onto the affected area. This procedure helps prevent regrowth of the pterygium. Another surgical option involves radiation therapy, which utilizes low doses of radiation to shrink the pterygium.

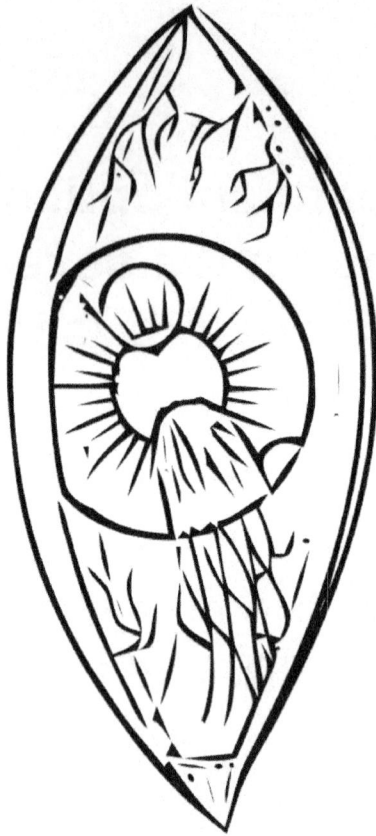

PTERYGIUM

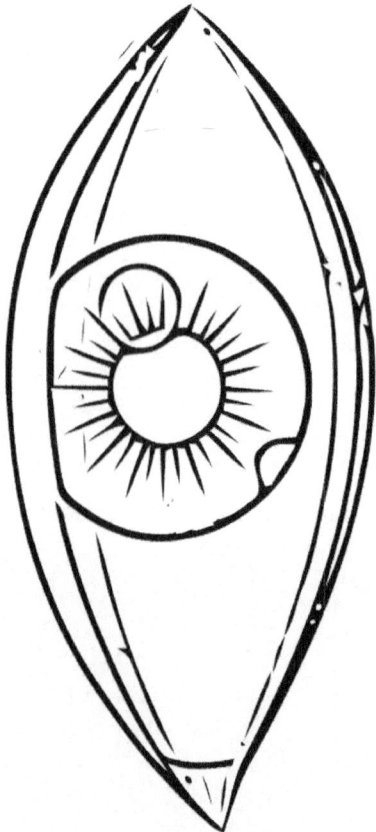

NORMAL EYE

100

Pinguecula

Pinguecula, a common eye condition that affects many individuals, particularly those who spend ample time outdoors, is characterized by the presence of a yellowish growth on the sclera, typically located near the corneal edge. Although it is generally not detrimental to ocular health, some patients may experience discomfort and irritation.

The precise cause of Pinguecula remains uncertain; however, experts believe that exposure to UV radiation from sunlight, wind, and dust plays a role. Additionally, factors such as age, dry eyes, and certain medications may contribute to its development. Notably, individuals residing in sunny regions or engaged in prolonged outdoor work are more susceptible to this condition.

Pinguecula usually appears as a yellowish or white bump on the conjunctiva, which is the clear tissue that covers the white part of the eye. It can occur on either side of the cornea and is typically located near the nose.

The growth may cause irritation, redness, and dryness in the affected eye. Patients may also experience a feeling of grittiness or foreign body sensation in the eye, especially when wearing contact lenses or exposed to windy conditions. In rare cases, pinguecula may grow large enough to affect vision or cause astigmatism.

There are multiple treatment options available for patients with Pinguecula. The primary treatment is the use of artificial tears, which can provide relief from dryness and irritation in the affected eye. Steroid eye drops may also be prescribed to diminish inflammation and swelling. In severe cases, surgery might be necessary to remove the growth if it is causing significant discomfort or vision issues.

A suitable alternative is utilizing protective eyewear like sunglasses or a wide-brimmed hat to shield the eyes against UV radiation and other environmental irritants. This not only helps prevent further growth of Pinguecula but also reduces symptoms. It is important to understand that while these treatments can prove effective, there is currently no known cure for Pinguecula, and it may reoccur even after treatment.

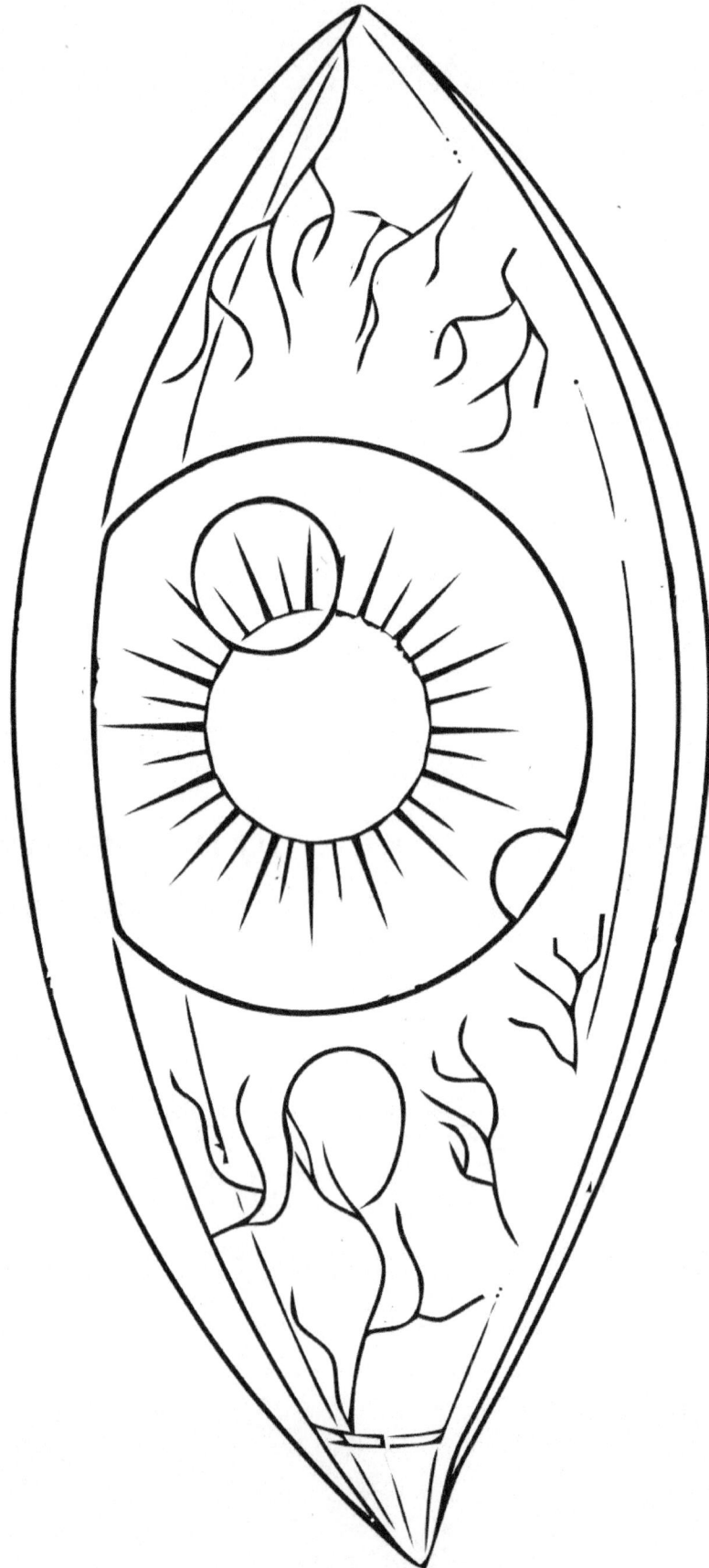

PINGUECULA

Ptosis

Ptosis is a medical condition that presents as the drooping of the upper eyelid, resulting in impaired vision. This condition can occur unilaterally or bilaterally at any stage of life. Various factors contribute to ptosis, including age, injury, muscle weakness, and nerve damage. Additionally, there are cases of congenital ptosis wherein individuals are born with this condition. While ptosis typically does not pose a threat to vision, it can have an impact on one's aesthetic appearance and self-esteem.

Ptosis

Ptosis, also known as drooping eyelid, is a condition that can impact either one or both eyes. The primary indication of ptosis is a visibly drooping eyelid, which can hinder clear vision. Additional symptoms may encompass eye fatigue, headaches, and strain on the eyebrows as the patient endeavors to compensate for the droopiness.

In more severe instances, ptosis has the potential to cause vision difficulties and potentially lead to amblyopia or lazy eye. If you are facing any of these symptoms, it is imperative to promptly seek medical attention in order to identify the underlying cause of your ptosis and receive appropriate treatment.

Ptosis

There are several factors that can contribute to the development of ptosis, including congenital defects, injury, aging, and neurological disorders. When ptosis is present from birth, it is known as congenital ptosis and is typically caused by a malfunctioning eyelid-lifting muscle. On the other hand, acquired ptosis can develop later in life due to factors such as injury, damage to the muscle or nerves, or various medical conditions. Neurological ptosis often occurs in conjunction with conditions like myasthenia gravis, which disrupts the muscles that control eye movement.

Regardless of its origin, ptosis can significantly impact an individual's quality of life by affecting their vision, appearance, and self-confidence. It is crucial to seek prompt medical attention if you suspect you may have ptosis because early diagnosis and treatment can help prevent further complications.

Ptosis

The process of diagnosing ptosis usually entails a thorough physical examination. This examination may encompass measuring the elevation of the eyelid, evaluating muscle strength, and assessing the patient's ocular mobility. Additionally, the doctor will gather a comprehensive medical history in order to ascertain if there are any potential underlying factors contributing to the ptosis.

Depending on the circumstances, further diagnostic tests may be required to validate the diagnosis or pinpoint the root cause of the ptosis. These additional evaluations might involve imaging tests like CT scans or MRIs, nerve conduction studies, or blood tests aimed at detecting specific medical conditions.

Ptosis

Treatment options for ptosis vary depending on the severity of the condition and its underlying cause. In cases where ptosis is impacting vision or causing discomfort, surgery is often recommended. During this procedure, the levator muscle responsible for eyelid movement is adjusted to restore a more natural position to the drooping eyelid. This surgery typically takes place under local anesthesia and can be performed as an outpatient procedure.

In some instances, medication may be prescribed to address ptosis, especially if it stems from a neurological disorder. Cholinesterase inhibitors are commonly used to enhance muscle strength and control, while botulinum toxin injections can temporarily paralyze the muscles involved in eyelid movement, thereby allowing for natural lifting of the eyelid.

Additionally, lifestyle changes like wearing glasses or using eye drops may be suggested to manage symptoms and promote overall eye health. With appropriate treatment options available, individuals experiencing ptosis can find relief and improve their quality of life.

Ptosis
of the upper eyelid

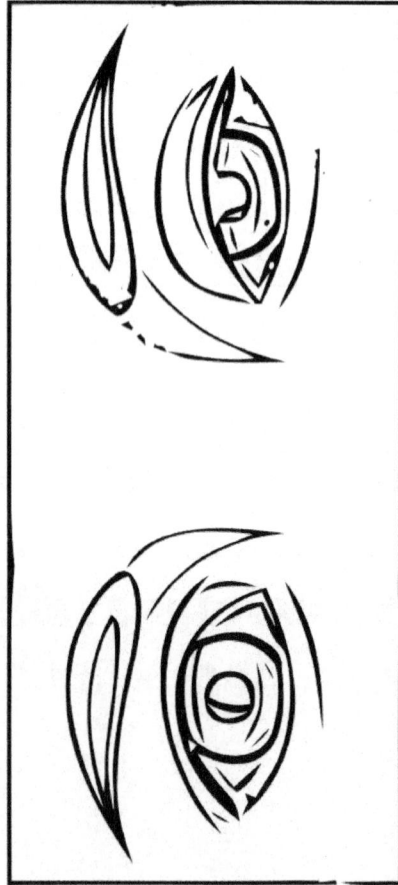

Ptosis in an adult

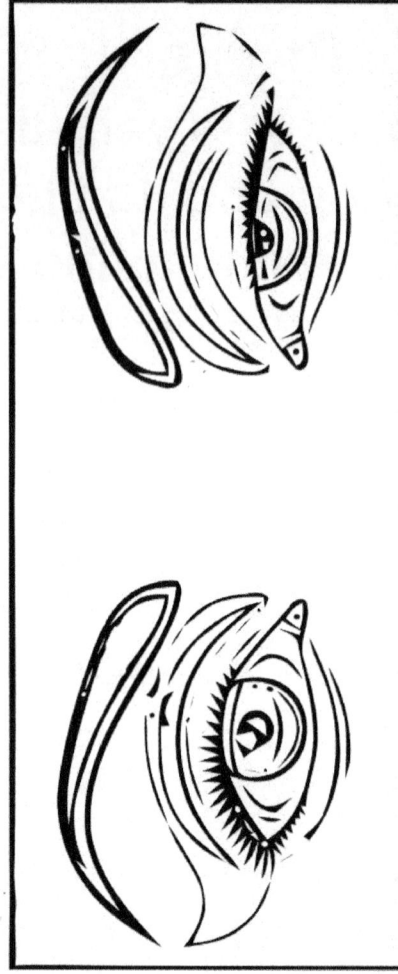

Ptosis in a child

Myopia

Myopia, also referred to as nearsightedness, is a prevalent vision condition that impacts a large number of individuals globally. This occurs when the eye is excessively long or when the cornea has excessive curvature, causing light to converge in front of the retina rather than on it. Consequently, distant objects appear blurred while close-up objects remain clear.

Individuals with myopia may encounter challenges in seeing objects at a distance, such as road signs or chalkboards, but have no difficulty seeing things up close, like books or computer screens. Fortunately, myopia can be successfully corrected through the use of glasses, contact lenses, or refractive surgery.

Based on current research findings, there has been a noticeable increase in the prevalence of myopia over the past few years. It is estimated that around 30% of the global population is now affected by this condition.

It is important to note that the prevalence of myopia can vary significantly across different age groups and geographical regions. For instance, countries like China and Singapore have reported much higher rates of myopia, with up to 80% of young adults being affected. On the other hand, regions such as Africa and South America have relatively lower prevalence rates.

Several factors can contribute to the development of myopia. Urban areas tend to have higher rates of myopia, possibly due to increased exposure to near-work activities and reduced outdoor time. Similarly, individuals who spend significant amounts of time engaged in activities that require close-up work may also be at a greater risk.

Myopia, also known as nearsightedness, is a common refractive error. It occurs when the eye is too long or the cornea is excessively curved, leading to the focus of light in front of the retina instead of on it. This condition causes blurry distance vision.

Although genetics play a significant role in the development of myopia, environmental factors can also contribute to its progression. Excessive screen time, lack of outdoor activity, and poor lighting are some examples of these factors. Additionally, lifestyle choices such as diet and physical activity may have an impact on myopia.

Myopia, also referred to as nearsightedness, is a visual impairment that causes distant objects to appear blurry while close objects remain clear. This condition often results in eye strain, headaches, and fatigue, particularly when engaging in activities like reading or driving.

In addition to blurred vision, individuals with myopia may experience squinting, reduced visibility at night, and the need to sit closer to screens. It's crucial to understand that the severity of these symptoms can vary depending on the extent of an individual's myopia.

The most commonly used treatment option for myopia is corrective lenses, such as glasses or contact lenses. These devices work by altering the path of light entering the eye, enhancing the clarity of images on the retina and improving overall vision.

Another treatment approach called orthokeratology involves wearing specialized contact lenses overnight that gently reshape the cornea, resulting in clear vision during waking hours without the need for corrective lenses. Orthokeratology is often recommended for individuals with mild to moderate myopia.

For more severe cases of myopia, refractive surgeries like LASIK or PRK can be considered. These surgical procedures involve using a laser to reshape the cornea, permanently enhancing visual acuity. However, it's important to note that refractive surgeries are typically reserved for patients with significant myopia.

Focal point

Myopia

Vitreous body

lens

Light

Central retinal artery

Optic nerve

Focal point

Choroid

Sclera

Central Retinal vein

Retina

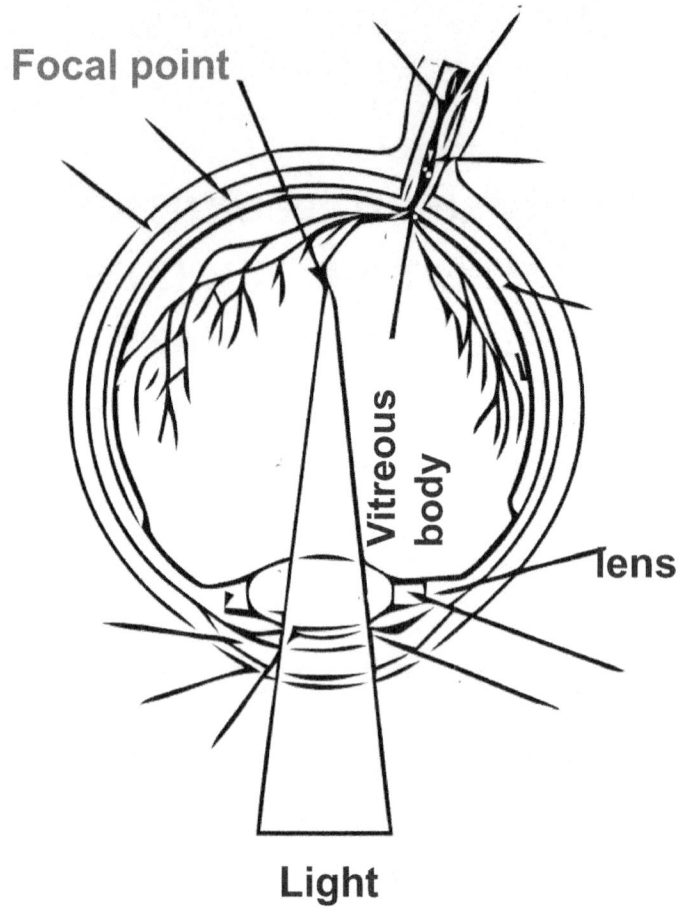

Normal vision

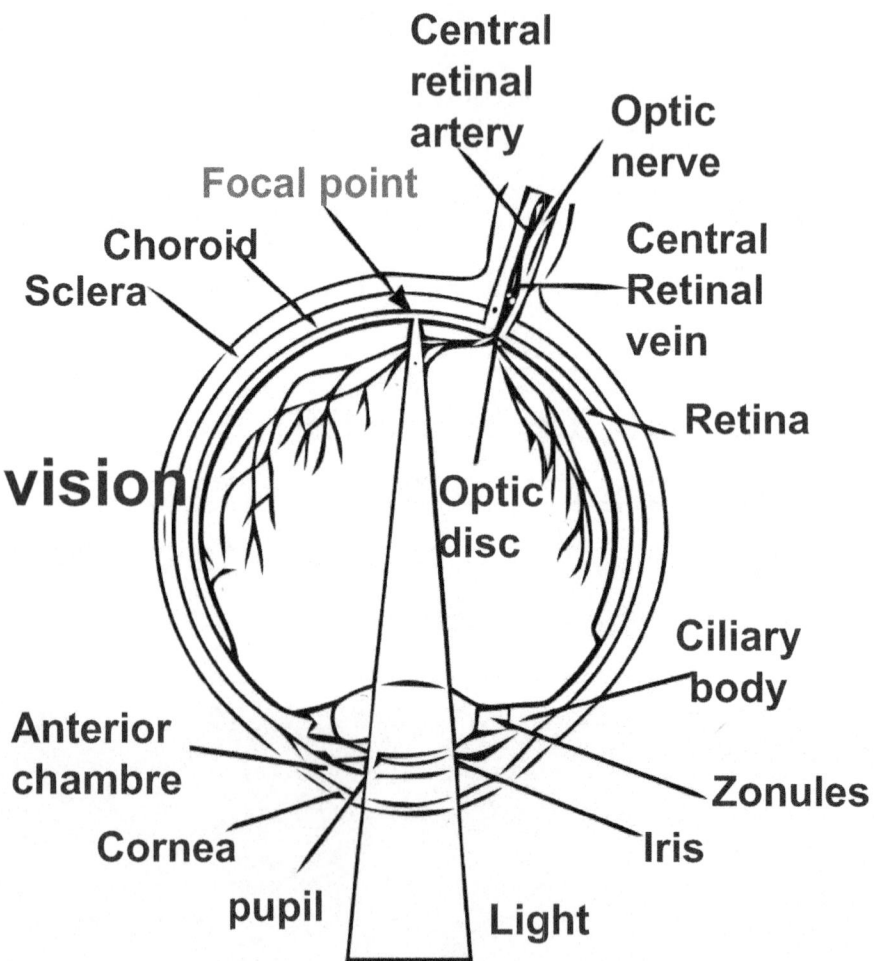

Optic disc

Ciliary body

Anterior chambre

Zonules

Cornea

Iris

pupil

Light

Myopia

The most commonly used treatment option for myopia is corrective lenses, such as glasses or contact lenses. These devices work by altering the path of light entering the eye, enhancing the clarity of images on the retina and improving overall vision.

Another treatment approach called orthokeratology involves wearing specialized contact lenses overnight that gently reshape the cornea, resulting in clear vision during waking hours without the need for corrective lenses. Orthokeratology is often recommended for individuals with mild to moderate myopia.

For more severe cases of myopia, refractive surgeries like LASIK or PRK can be considered. These surgical procedures involve using a laser to reshape the cornea, permanently enhancing visual acuity. However, it's important to note that refractive surgeries are typically reserved for patients with significant myopia.

LASIK Surgery for Myopia

Before

Cornea

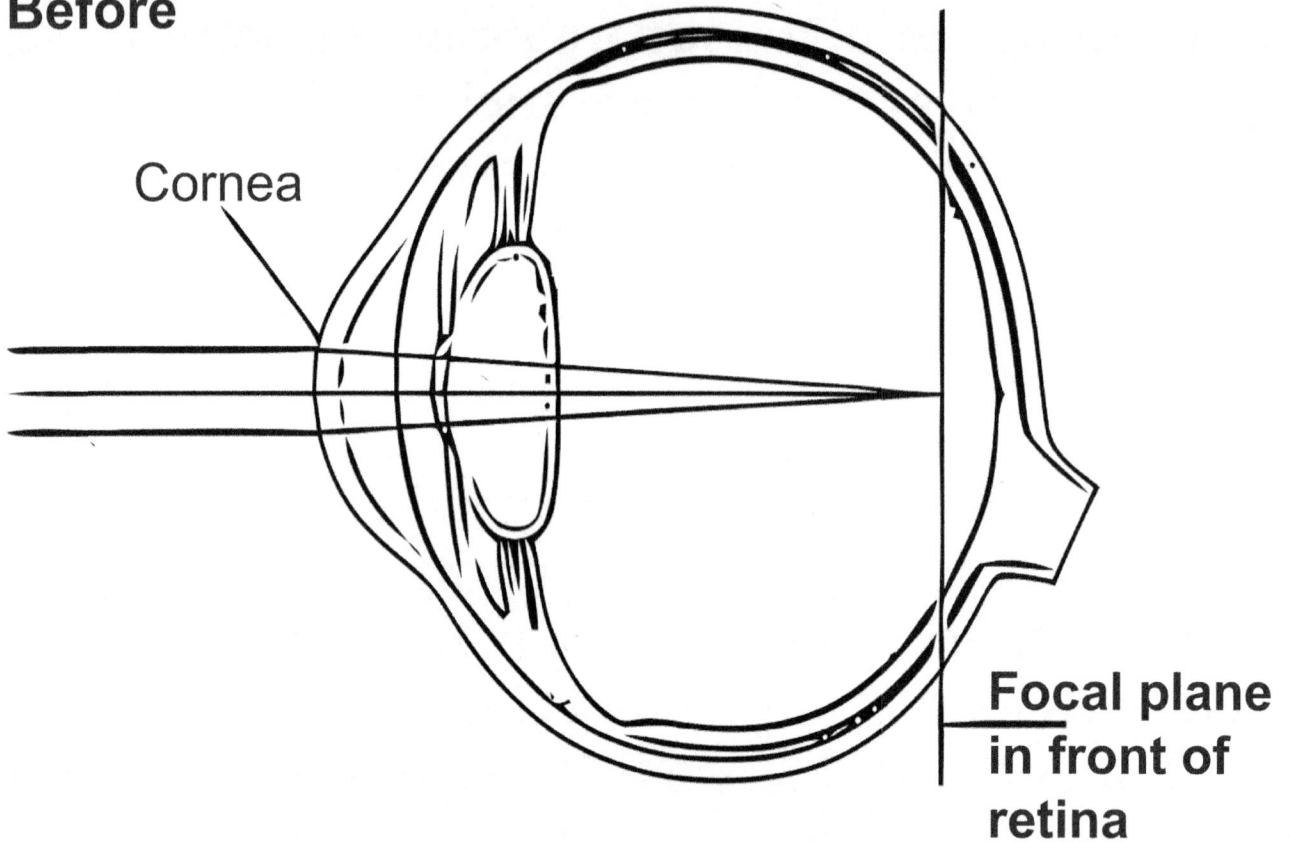

Focal plane in front of retina

After

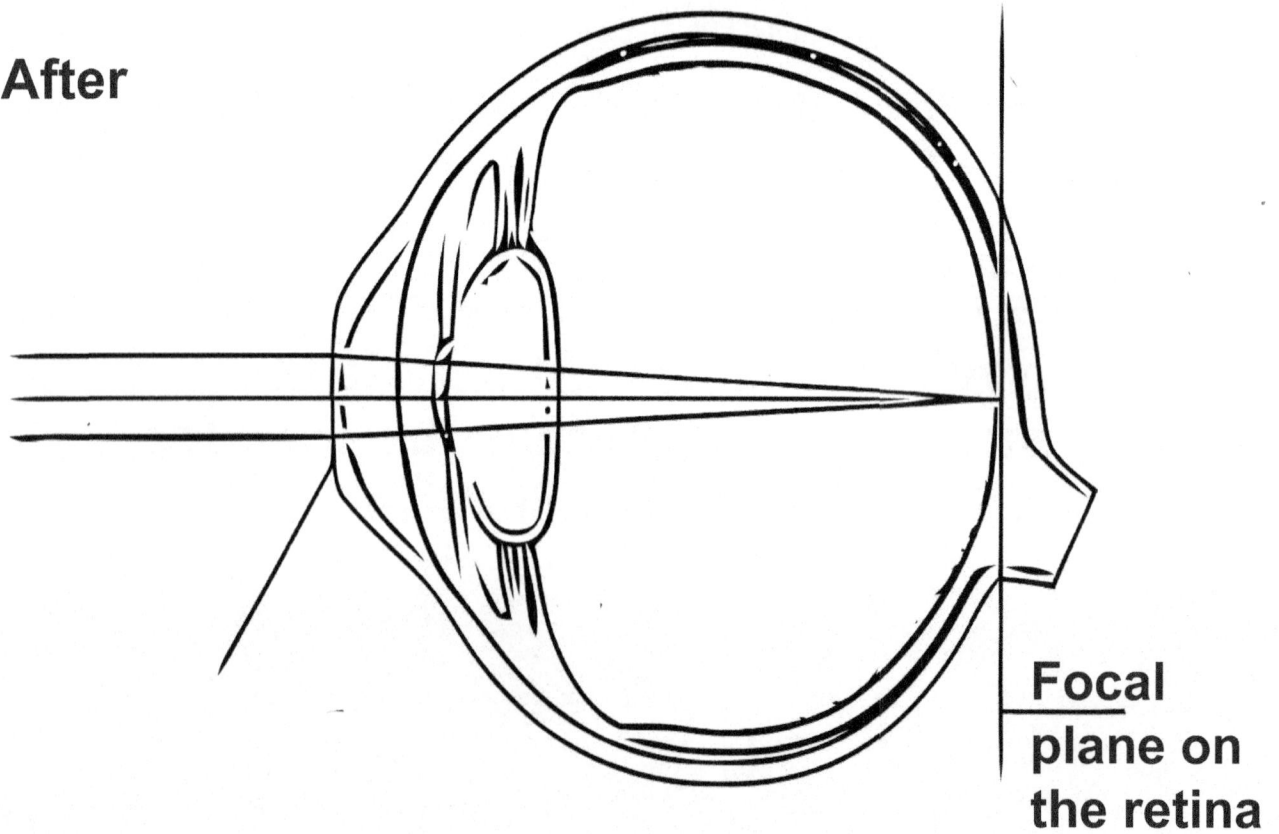

Focal plane on the retina

Hyperopia

Hyperopia, also referred to as farsightedness, is a prevalent refractive error that impacts a significant number of individuals across the globe. This condition arises when the eye is shorter than average or when the cornea lacks sufficient curvature, resulting in light focusing behind the retina rather than directly on it.

It is worth noting that hyperopia tends to be more common among younger individuals and generally diminishes with age, as highlighted by the American Optometric Association.

Hyperopia

Hyperopia, or farsightedness, is a prevalent refractive error that affects a significant number of individuals globally. This condition occurs when light entering the eye is focused behind the retina instead of directly on it, resulting in distant objects appearing clearer than those up close.

In contrast to myopia, which is nearsightedness, hyperopia leads to difficulties in seeing nearby objects while maintaining clear vision of distant ones. Additionally, hyperopia can cause eye strain, headaches, and fatigue—particularly after prolonged periods of reading or computer use. To ensure early detection and effective management of hyperopia, it is crucial to schedule regular eye examinations.

Hyperopia

Hyperopia, a prevalent refractive error, impacts numerous individuals globally. Though the precise cause of hyperopia remains partially uncertain, several factors play a role in its development.

Genetics stands among the primary causes of hyperopia. When one or both parents possess hyperopia, their children have an increased likelihood of acquiring it. Other elements that can contribute to hyperopia encompass specific medical conditions like diabetes, as well as environmental factors such as prolonged periods of reading or computer use.

Symptoms of Hyperopia

Hyperopia, also known as farsightedness, is a refractive error that makes it difficult to see objects up close. People with hyperopia may experience eye strain or headaches when trying to read or focus on nearby objects.

In addition to difficulty seeing up close, hyperopia can also cause problems with depth perception and make it harder to see in low light conditions. For example, driving at night may be more challenging for someone with hyperopia.

Diagnosis and Treatment

Hyperopia, also known as farsightedness, is a common refractive error that affects many people. It occurs when the eye is too short or the cornea is too flat, causing light to focus behind the retina instead of directly on it.

Diagnosis of hyperopia involves a comprehensive eye exam, which includes visual acuity testing and a refraction test. Treatment options for hyperopia include glasses, contact lenses, and surgery. Glasses and contact lenses work by refracting light to compensate for the shape of the eye, while surgery can reshape the cornea to improve vision.

Hyperopia

Focal point

Vitreous body

lens

Light

Central retinal artery

Focal point

Optic nerve

Central Retinal vein

Choroid

Sclera

Retina

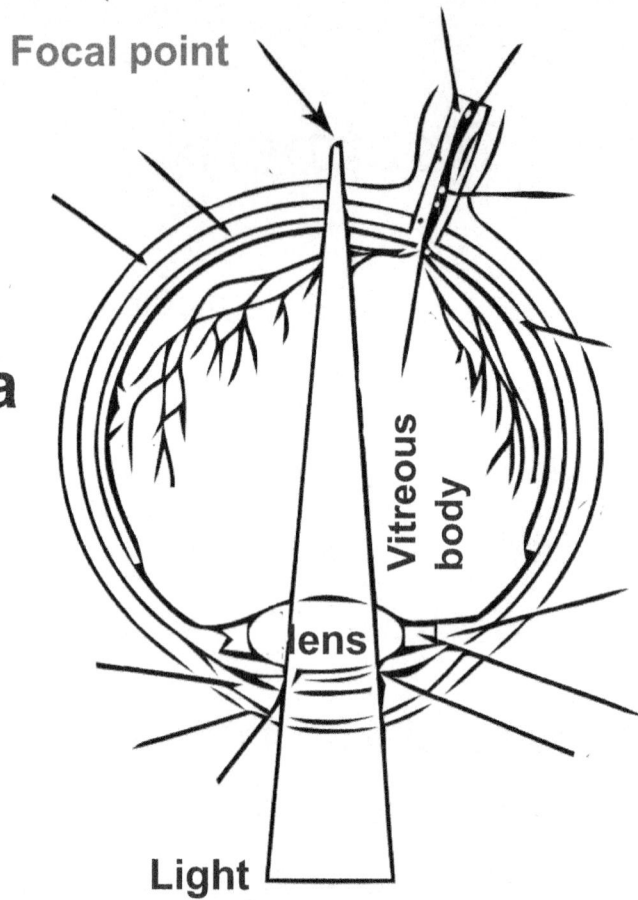

Normal vision

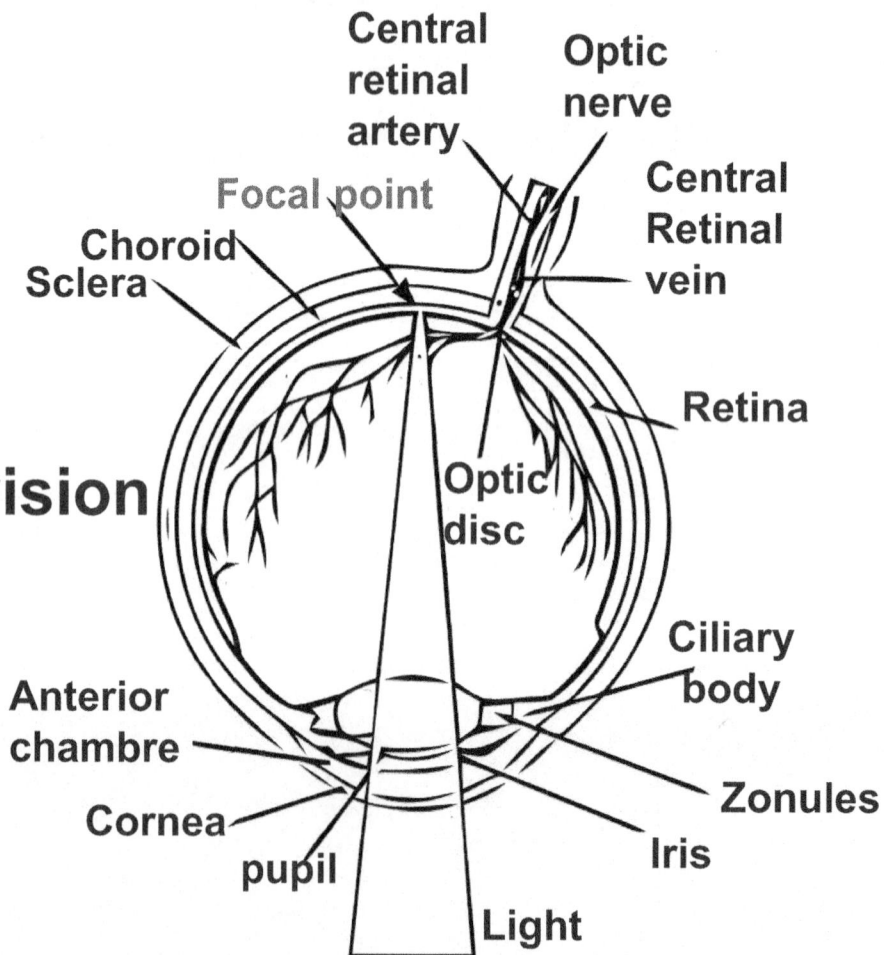

Optic disc

Ciliary body

Anterior chambre

Zonules

Cornea

Iris

pupil

Light

Astigmatism

Astigmatism is a common eye condition that affects millions of people worldwide. It occurs when the cornea or lens of the eye is not perfectly round, causing blurred vision at all distances. This can make it difficult to see clearly and perform everyday tasks such as reading, driving, and watching television.

While astigmatism can be frustrating, it is important to remember that it is a treatable condition. With the right care and attention, most people with astigmatism can enjoy clear vision and an improved quality of life.

Symptoms of Astigmatism

One of the most common symptoms of astigmatism is blurry vision. This can make it difficult to see objects clearly, especially at a distance. For example, you may have trouble reading street signs or recognizing faces from across the room. Blurry vision can also make it hard to focus on details, which can be frustrating and tiring.

Another common symptom is eye strain. This occurs when your eyes have to work harder than usual to focus on objects due to the irregular shape of the cornea or lens. Eye strain can cause discomfort, fatigue, and even headaches. For example, if you spend a lot of time looking at a computer screen or reading small print, you may experience eye strain more frequently.

Causes of Astigmatism

Astigmatism is a common vision condition that occurs when the cornea or lens of the eye has an irregular shape. This can cause light to be refracted unevenly, resulting in blurry or distorted vision. There are several different causes of astigmatism, including genetics, eye injuries, and certain medical conditions. In some cases, astigmatism may be present at birth or develop during childhood.

One of the most common causes of astigmatism is genetics. If one or both parents have astigmatism, their children are more likely to develop the condition. Eye injuries, such as a blunt trauma or penetrating injury, can also cause astigmatism. Certain medical conditions, such as keratoconus or corneal scarring, can also lead to astigmatism. Additionally, some surgeries, such as cataract surgery, can cause astigmatism as a side effect.

Diagnosing Astigmatism

Astigmatism is a common condition that affects the way light enters the eye, causing blurry or distorted vision. If you are experiencing symptoms such as headaches, eye strain, or difficulty seeing clearly, it is important to schedule an eye exam with your optometrist or ophthalmologist.

During the exam, your eye doctor will perform a series of tests to determine if you have astigmatism. These may include a visual acuity test, which measures how well you can see at various distances, and a keratometry test, which measures the curvature of your cornea. Your doctor may also use a phoropter to determine the best prescription for corrective lenses, if needed.

Treating Astigmatism

Astigmatism is a common condition that affects the way light enters the eye, causing blurry or distorted vision. Fortunately, there are several treatment options available to correct astigmatism and improve vision.

One option is corrective lenses, such as glasses or contact lenses, which can help to refocus light entering the eye. However, these lenses may need to be adjusted periodically as the shape of the eye changes over time. Another option is LASIK surgery, which involves reshaping the cornea to correct vision. While this procedure can be highly effective, it also carries some risks and may not be suitable for everyone. A third option is orthokeratology, which involves wearing special contact lenses overnight to reshape the cornea. This can provide temporary relief from astigmatism, but may not be a permanent solution.

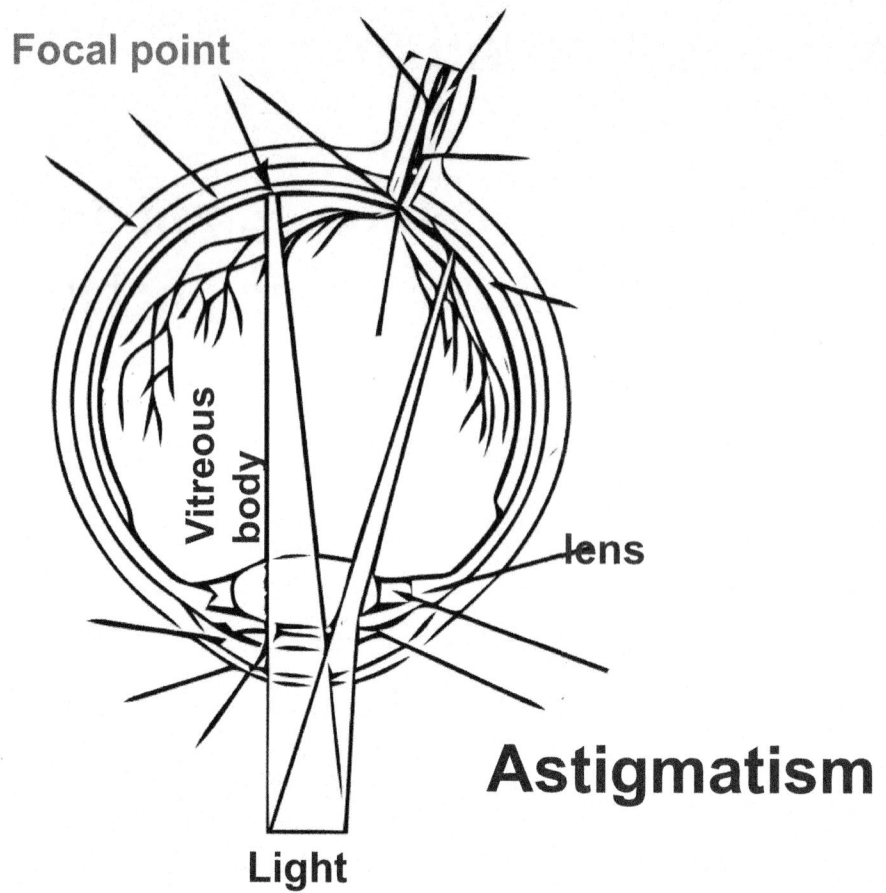

Focal point

Vitreous body

lens

Astigmatism

Light

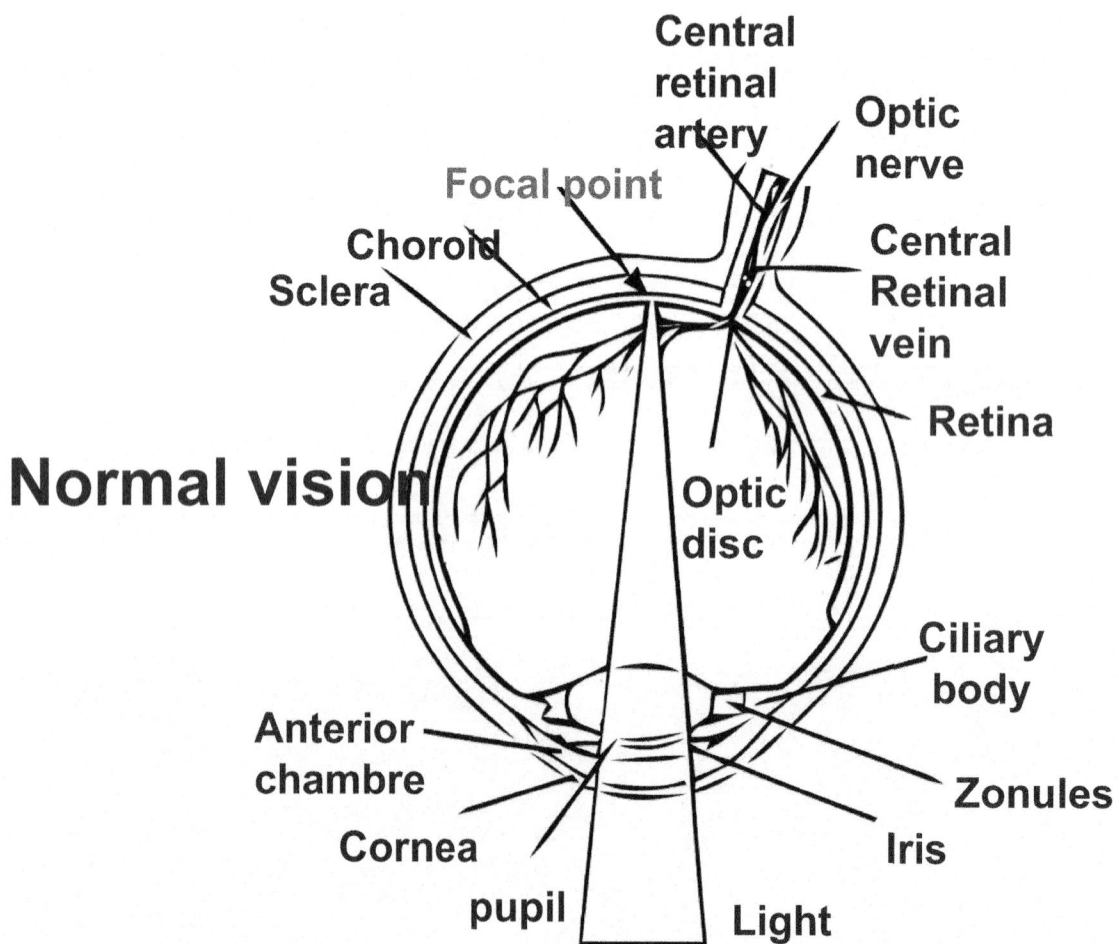

Central retinal artery

Optic nerve

Focal point

Central Retinal vein

Choroid

Sclera

Retina

Normal vision

Optic disc

Ciliary body

Anterior chambre

Zonules

Cornea

Iris

pupil

Light

130

Printed in Great Britain
by Amazon